Neurosurgery

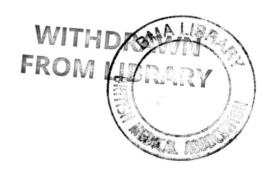
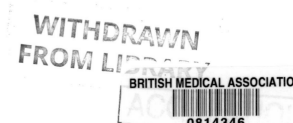

Neurosurgery

The Essential Guide to the Oral and Clinical Neurosurgical Examination

Vivian A. Elwell BA Hons., MA (Cantab), MBBS, MRCS, FRCS (Neuro.Surg)
Central London Senior Spinal Fellow, The National Hospital for Neurology and Neurosurgery, Queen Square, London, UK

Ramez Kirollos MBChB, MD, FRCS (Ed), FRCS (Eng), FRCS (Neuro.Surg), European Certificate of Neurosurgery
Consultant Neurosurgeon, Addenbrooke's Hospital, Cambridge, UK

Syed Al-Haddad MB BCh BAO (NUI), MSc (Trauma), MRCS, FRCS (Neuro.Surg)
Consultant Neurosurgeon, Aberdeen Royal Infirmary, Aberdeen, Scotland

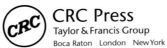
CRC Press
Taylor & Francis Group
Boca Raton   London   New York

CRC Press is an imprint of the
Taylor & Francis Group, an **informa** business

CRC Press
Taylor & Francis Group
6000 Broken Sound Parkway NW, Suite 300
Boca Raton, FL 33487-2742

© 2015 by Taylor & Francis Group, LLC
CRC Press is an imprint of Taylor & Francis Group, an Informa business

No claim to original U.S. Government works

Printed on acid-free paper
Version Date: 20140908

International Standard Book Number-13: 978-1-4822-2760-4 (Paperback)

Visit the Taylor & Francis Web site at
http://www.taylorandfrancis.com

and the CRC Press Web site at
http://www.crcpress.com

Dedication

This book is dedicated to all past, present and future neurosurgical patients.

The capacity of man himself is only revealed when, under stress and responsibility, he breaks through his educational shell, and he may then be a splendid surprise to himself no less than to this teachers.

Harvey Cushing (1869–1939)

Contents

About the Authors

Vivian A. Elwell BA Hons., MA (Cantab), MBBS, MRCS, FRCS (Neuro.Surg)

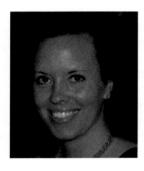

Having completed her specialist registrar neurosurgery run-through training in London, Miss Elwell is currently working as a Post-CCT Senior Spinal Fellow. She has held posts in Accident and Emergency, Orthopaedics, Neurosurgery, and General Surgery within the Surgical Rotation at St Mary's Hospital, Imperial College Healthcare NHS Trust, London.

Miss Elwell's awards include the Swinford Edward Silver Medal Prize for her OSCE Examination; the Columbia University Research Fellowship at Columbia College of Physicians and Surgeons in New York City, USA; the Columbia University King's Crown Gold and Silver Medal Awards; the Kathrine Dulin Folger Cancer Research Fellowship and the 'Who's Who Young Scientists Award'. In 2010, Miss Elwell was a finalist for the BMA's Junior Doctor of the Year Award.

Miss Elwell earned a Bachelor's Degree in Biological Sciences at Columbia College, Columbia University, and a Master of Arts degree from the University of Cambridge. She earned a Bachelor of Medicine and Bachelor of Surgery from the Imperial College School of Medicine. She is a Fellow of the Royal College of Surgeons.

Ramez Kirollos MBChB, MD, FRCS (Ed), FRCS (Eng), FRCS (Neuro.Surg), European Certificate of Neurosurgery

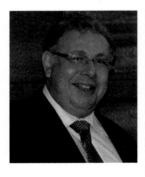

Mr Kirollos graduated from the Medical School at the University of Alexandria, Egypt, in 1984. In 1987, he pursued his post-graduate medical education in the UK. He was awarded the Hallett prize by the Royal College of Surgeons of England for the results of his primary FRCS examination. Mr Kirollos trained in neurosurgery at the Atkinson Morley Hospital in London, the Frenchay Hospital in Bristol, the Leeds General Infirmary, and the Walton Centre for Neurology and Neurosurgery in Liverpool. He obtained an MD degree for his research into photodynamic therapy of pituitary adenomas. Mr Kirollos completed a skull base fellowship under Dr Gentili at the Toronto Western Hospital. In 2001, he was appointed Consultant Neurosurgeon at Addenbrooke's Hospital in Cambridge. His main clinical interests include anterior and middle skull base, pituitary and pineal surgery, and surgical treatment of arteriovenous malformations.

A passion for neurosurgical technique based on the thorough understanding of anatomy has accompanied Mr Kirollos' neurosurgical training and forms the basis of his surgical practice. He keenly shares this philosophy and knowledge with his trainees. Mr Kirollos has been actively involved in day-to-day teaching of medical students and junior and middle-grade neurosurgical trainees. He oversees weekly registrar teaching sessions at Addenbrooke's Hospital. Mr Kirollos serve on the faculty for Neuroanatomy of Operative Approaches and the British Neurosurgical Trainee courses since their conception in 2005 and 2010, respectively. In 2006, Mr Kirollos was elected as a member of the Court of Examiners of the Royal College of Surgeons of England. In 2010, for his commitment to surgical education, he received the prestigious Silver Scalpel Award. He is the chairman of the British Neurovascular Group (2013–2015).

Syed Abdullah Al-Haddad MB BCh BAO (NUI), MSc (Trauma), MRCS, FRCS (Neuro. Surg)

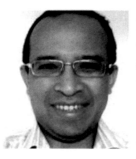

Mr Al-Haddad is originally from Malaysia, where he studied and won the Most Outstanding Student Award from the Royal Military College. Subsequently, he was awarded a full scholarship to study medicine in the UK. During his undergraduate years he excelled in both academic and extracurricular activities. He represented his college at the intervarsity level in rugby, hockey and volleyball. He was nominated as the sportsman of the year and won the Barker Anatomy Prize. He graduated from the Royal College of Surgeons in Ireland in 1996.

He went on to complete a Master's degree at the University of Birmingham in 2000 in the study of surgical outcome of depressed skull fractures. He commenced his neurosurgical training at the Walton Centre in Liverpool, where he developed his interest in neuro-oncology research. He undertook further training in neurosurgery in Manchester, Leeds, Aberdeen and Edinburgh before being appointed a Consultant Neurosurgeon in Aberdeen, Scotland. Throughout, he has been actively involved in teaching both undergraduate and postgraduate students. He is a faculty member for Leeds and Edinburgh operative neuroanatomy courses. He has published numerous articles in peer-reviewed journals and also contributed a section on the online neuroscience module (www.ebrainjnc.com).

Mr Al-Haddad is the founder and director of the highly successful Aberdeen FRCS (SN) viva course. The course has run twice a year since 2010, with the emphasis on giving practical advice to produce outstanding neurosurgeons who are well prepared for the challenge of the neurosurgical exam.

Acknowledgements

We would like to thank our colleagues, family and friends. This book would not have been possible without the ongoing support and encouragement of the following people:

Miss Elwell: Mrs Carole D Elwell, Mr and Mrs John A Cervieri Jr, Dr and Mrs George Leib, Mr Laurence Watkins and Mr David Choi.

Mr Kirollos: The inspiration of my late parents Dr Wadie Kirollos and Mrs Dalal Mikhael, the support of my wife Nivine and sons Karim and Sherif.

Mr Al-Haddad: Mr Syed Mohamed Al-Haddad, Mrs Rabiah bt Othman, Munirah Aljoofre, Khadijah, Alwi, Zainab and Mohamed, Osman, Ading, Aman, Intan and Hussein Al-Haddad.

Contributors

Dr Nabeel S Alshafai
Complex Spine Fellow, University of Toronto, Canada
Director of the Comprehensive Clinical Neurosurgery Review Course
American Board of Neurologic Surgery (ABNS)
Royal College of Physicians and Surgeons of Canada (FRCSC)
European Association of Neurosurgical Societies (EANS)
Introduction

Mr Nicholas DP Hall
Senior Clinical Fellow, Addenbrooke's Hospital, Cambridge, UK
Royal Australasian College of Surgeons
Introduction

Mr Bedansh Roy Chaudhary
Specialist Registrar in Neurosurgery, Addenbrooke's Hospital, Cambridge, UK
Chapter 1: How to succeed

Mr Ravi Vashu
Specialist Registrar in Neurosurgery, Aberdeen Royal Infirmary, Aberdeen, Scotland, UK
*Chapter 5: The viva: investigation of the neurosurgical patient including neuroradiology and
    neuropathology*

Dr Alan Forster
Consultant Neurophysiologist, Aberdeen Royal Infirmary, Aberdeen, Scotland, UK
*Chapter 5: The viva: investigation of the neurosurgical patient including neuroradiology and
    neuropathology*

Foreword

When I took the final FRCS exam in 1974, I had been working a 1:2 rota as a young registrar in general surgery, commuting from Glasgow to Falkirk. I had completed 18 months as a senior house officer and research assistant in neurosurgery with a paper in *Nature New Biology*. In London, the examiner asked me what specialty I wished to follow. On hearing that I was a fledgling neurosurgeon, he asked me to tell him what I knew about haemorrhoids.

'Plus ça change, plus c'est la même chose'.

Two weeks later I had better luck in Edinburgh. Shortly thereafter, I was on the plane to Philadelphia for my research fellowship. Stress, what stress?

Examinations are a necessary evil. Necessary because they provide an independent assurance to patients, families, the general public, employers, defence organizations, the General Medical Council, future colleagues and all grades of staff that the successful candidate has acquired a basic core of knowledge and has displayed the ability to use it, albeit in the artificial environment of the examination hall. It is one important hurdle in the completion of training that indicates that the candidate is probably safe and has the flexibility of mind to cope with the ever-changing understanding of and technology within his or her specialty. 'Evil' because too many examinations and assessments can stultify, regiment thought and delay the development of lateral thinking and initiative.

However, like life, examinations can sometimes be unfair. As George Cruikshank's cartoon from 1811 illustrates, there was a time when examiners could be capricious in their judgement. There are now many checks and balances to reduce the risk of such errant behaviour. It is only right that examinations should be professionally organized and transparent in what is expected. Examinees in school and university

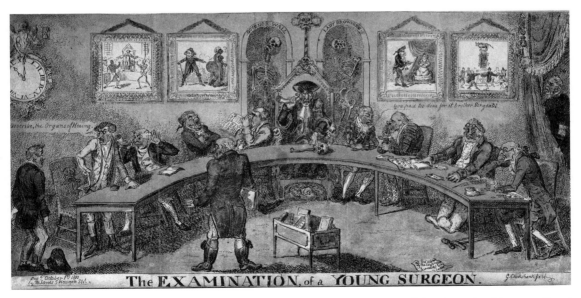

The Examination of a Young Surgeon by George Cruikshank, 1811. Courtesy of the Hunterian Museum, Royal College of Surgeons of England, London, UK.

have little else to think about. Trainee surgeons in their early 30s have patient care, research projects, families and mortgages to distract them.

There are occasions when an otherwise clinically competent candidate underperforms. This admirable and concise handbook provides invaluable insight and advice on how to prepare for the oral and clinical parts of neurosurgery examinations and reduce the risk of failure. The authors, including one who won the Silver Scalpel Award for his many contributions to neurosurgery training in the UK, are to be congratulated on their initiative, insight and compassion.

Professor John Pickard
Former Chairman of Examiners
Intercollegiate Examination in Surgical Neurology
Addenbrooke's Hospital, Cambridge, UK

Testimonial

Neurosurgery is a fast-moving, exciting specialty that demands much from trainees and established clinicians alike. Good technical skill goes without saying, but perhaps more important are sound knowledge, clear thinking and quick decision making. Recognizing unusual conditions and pertinent warning signs, anticipating complications, and deciding when not to operate are paramount.

This book reviews the basic science and concepts required to pass the Royal College of Surgeons of England final examination in neurosurgery. It builds on these foundations to explain the nature of good clinical practice in neurosurgery, with clinical scenarios to illustrate key concepts. Unlike many other texts available, it is focused on equipping the candidate not only to pass an examination, but also to pass beyond into clinical practise. The book is not an end-point in itself, but a beginning, to stimulate the reader into thinking about and discussing clinical neurosurgery from theory to practice. It is important that candidates practise short cases, long cases, and *viva voce* examination. Repetitive practice will reinforce learning and boost confidence. Often candidates fail not because of lack of knowledge, but rather because of poor confidence, which translates into weak delivery and hesitant performance. This book will not replace bedside teaching and practice but will stimulate the candidate to engage in neurosurgical thought and decision making.

To prepare for short and long cases, it is important for the candidate to practise examination technique on normal individuals (spouses, fellow residents, medical students) as well as patients. By repeatedly examining normal subjects, the candidate will improve fluency of technique and develop confidence and professionalism. By examining patients, the candidate will acquire diagnostic skills, become accustomed to real-life situations, and develop a courteous and considerate patient manner. The doctor who wins the patient's confidence will elicit the symptoms and signs that are required to make a correct diagnosis.

To prepare for the *viva voce* examination, the candidate should be quizzed regularly by colleagues or senior surgeons, to experience the adrenaline rush of being 'put on the spot' and to become accustomed to answering questions under pressure. This book can be used as a starting point for discussions, to remind the examinee of the breadth of the neurosurgical syllabus and provide material for *viva voce* practice.

Good clinical practice revolves around sound theoretical and practical knowledge, clinical experience, and examination preparation. Awareness of research methodology and techniques of literature review, statistics and interpretation will allow the reader to critically appraise the pieces of evidence that influence clinical practice today. The key to becoming a competent neurosurgeon is practice, practice, practice. After acquiring the basic knowledge and skills required, continued exposure to patients and operating theatres will consolidate experience. It is obvious when a candidate has had little clinical exposure, and therefore it is important for residents not to attempt an examination too early in their training. Experience comes with spending time on the wards and in the operating theatre, and there is no fast-track way of learning neurosurgery. Like all apprenticeships, improvement takes time, and there are no short-cuts. Like learning to fly an airplane, the number of hours at the controls is important. But this book allows the reader to consolidate the experience gained during a neurosurgical apprenticeship and to fine-tune the knowledge that the resident has already acquired over the years. It allows the resident to pass the examination and begin a fulfilling career in neurosurgery.

And then the hard work really begins!

Mr David Choi MA, MBChB, FRCS(SN), PhD
Reader in Neurosurgery
University College London
Institute of Neurology

Honorary Consultant Neurosurgeon
The National Hospital for Neurology and Neurosurgery
Queen Square, London, UK

Preface

Neurosurgery: The Essential Guide to the Oral and Clinical Neurosurgical Examination provides a concise, logical and practical guidebook of core knowledge and principles for the neurosurgical clinical examination.

Because you have passed the written neurosurgical examination, you have demonstrated that you have the required knowledge. Now, your written knowledge must be translated into an oral format in a safe, organized and non-intimidating manner. The main purpose of this examination is to ensure that you are a safe and competent neurosurgeon.

The viva examination ensures that the candidate understands the essential knowledge, rather than having detailed knowledge of selected topics. Success is seen once you place yourself in the examiner's shoes. During the examination, there should be a variety of topics discussed within an allocated time period. It cannot be overemphasized that you should tailor your answers to the allocated time. For example, if the time allocated is 10 minutes to cover three topics, your answer for each topic should be 3 minutes in duration and include the salient points. Therefore, for each topic, a minimum of three key points should be presented. During your final preparation, ensure that you have memorized the key points for the topics mentioned in the syllabus, rather than reading new material.

This book is designed to guide candidates preparing for the International and Intercollegiate FRCS Specialty Examination in Neurosurgery. It will also help prepare for the American Board of Neurological Surgery (ABNS) and other neurosurgical examinations around the world.

The Intercollegiate FRCS (Section II) examination is the clinical component of the examination and consists of a series of carefully designed and structured interviews on clinical topics. The examination syllabus, format and content are common to The Royal College of Surgeons of Edinburgh, The Royal College of Surgeons of England, The Royal College of Physicians and Surgeons of Glasgow and The Royal College of Surgeons in Ireland. This examination is designed and set by the Royal Colleges to assess the knowledge, skills and attributes acquired during neurosurgical training. The Section II examination is 2 hours and 30 minutes long and is taken over two days. On the first day, the examination comprises long and short cases. The long cases test the candidate's structured and logical approach to history taking and clinical examination. In addition, the candidate needs to formulate a list of differential diagnoses, interpret the appropriate investigations, and provide a clear management plan. The short cases test the candidate's clinical knowledge, diagnostic acumen, investigation and interpretation, and treatment options. Overall, the themes of history taking, breaking bad news, professionalism, and medical ethics are assessed while the candidate demonstrates clear reasoning and judgement. The viva is held on the second day and is divided into the following sections: operative surgery and surgical anatomy; investigation of the neurosurgical patient including neuroradiology; and non-operative clinical practice and neurosurgery.

We have written this book in conjunction with the Aberdeen FRCS (SN) viva courses, which help trainees identify high-yield topics for the neurosurgical examination, target the candidate's strengths and identify areas of potential weakness.

This book is based on our own clinical practice, teaching and examination experiences. It provides a greater understanding of neuroscience and the ability to solve problems under pressure. This book guides you through the neurosurgical examination and will be invaluable in your future surgical practice but is not a replacement for neurosurgical textbooks and practical experience.

We wish you the best of luck in your future career!

Vivian A Elwell
Ramez Kirollos
Syed Al-Haddad

Introduction

Intercollegiate Specialty Examination in Neurosurgery (UK)

The intercollegiate surgical curriculum provides the framework for neurosurgical training in the UK. It provides the neurosurgical syllabus and establishes the required standards for completion of training. While coupling basic and applied clinical neuroscience, the major areas of neurosurgical specialist interest are paediatric neurosurgery, neuro-oncology, functional neurosurgery, neurovascular surgery, skull base surgery, spinal surgery and traumatology. Current advances in microsurgical techniques, non-invasive imaging, neuro-anaesthesia, intensive care and image-guided surgery, as well as the introduction of radio-oncological and interventional treatment, are now incorporated into training. This book provides a template for the neurosurgical examination in line with the recognized standard defined by the Examination Board.

The structured clinical examination has the advantage of sampling the curriculum while allowing the examiners to observe the candidate's clinical ability and communication skills. During the long case, the trainee spends a fixed period of time with a patient to obtain a clinical history and perform a clinical examination. The examiners then assess the trainee by means of questions based on the patient's clinical symptoms and signs. During the short cases, two examiners assess your neurological examination skills. The examination assesses the candidate's professional capability, knowledge, judgement and communication skills.

The official scoring sheet provided by the Examination Board

Intercollegiate Specialty Boards Marking Descriptors

Rating Scale	Overall Professional Capability / Patient Care					Knowledge and Judgement			Quality of Response		'Bedside Manner'
	Personal qualities	Professionalism and ethics	Surgical experience	Adaptability to stress	Ability to deal with grey areas	Knowledge	Ability to justify	Clinical reasoning	Communication skills	Organisation and logical thought process	Applicable to Clinicals with patients
4	• The candidate demonstrated incompetence in the diagnosis and clinical management of patients to a level which caused serious concerns to the examiner					• Did not get beyond default questions • Failed in most/all competencies • Poor basic knowledge/ judgement/ understanding to a level of concern • Serious lack of knowledge			• Q: Does not get beyond default questions • A: Disorganized/ confused/ inconsistent answers, lacking insight • P: Un-persuadable- prompts do not work		• Abrupt/brusque manner • Arrogant • Inappropriate attitude/behaviour • No empathy • Rough handling of patients • Totally inappropriate examination of opposite sex
5	• The candidate failed to demonstrate competence in the diagnosis and clinical management of patients					• Demonstrated a lack of understanding • Difficulty in prioritizing • Gaps in knowledge • Poor deductive skills • Poor higher order thinking • Significant errors • Struggled to apply knowledge/ judgement/ management • Variable performance			• Q: Frequent use of default questions • A: Confused/ disorganized answers; hesitant and indecisive • P: Required frequent prompting		• Does not listen – patronizing • No introduction • Unsympathetic • Unobservant of body language

6	• The candidate demonstrated competence in the diagnosis and clinical management of patients	• Good knowledge and judgement of common problems • Important points mentioned • Instills confidence • No major errors	• Q: Copes with competence questions • A: Methodical approach to answers; has insight • P: Requires minimal prompting	• Appropriate exam of opposite sex • Considerate handling • Observes patient expression • Respects all • Responds to patient • Treats 'all' patients appropriately
7	• The candidate demonstrated confidence and competence in the diagnosis and clinical management of patients	• Ability to prioritize • Coped with difficult topics/problems • Good decision making/provided supporting evidence • Reached a good level of higher order thinking • Strong interpretation/ judgement but didn't quote the literature	• Q: Goes beyond the competence questions • A: Logical answers and provided good supporting reasons for answers • P: Fluent responses without prompting, but some prompting on literature	• Gains patient confidence quickly • Good awareness of patient's reaction • Puts patient at ease quickly
8	• The candidate demonstrated confidence and competence in the diagnosis and clinical management of patients to a level which would inspire confidence in the patient	• At ease with higher order thinking • Flawless knowledge plus insight and judgement • Good understanding/ knowledge/ management/ prioritization of complex issues • Had an understanding of the breadth and depth of the topic, and quoted from literature • High flyer • Strong interpretation/ judgement	• Q: Stretches examiners - answers questions at advanced level • A: Confident, clear, logical and focused answers • P: No prompting necessary	• Acts/talks at patient's level • Instills confidence in patient/rapport very good

Q: questions   A: answers   P: prompting.

American Board of Neurological Surgery

This examination is composed of a written and an oral component. The oral component is explained below.

- The examination lasts 3 hours and is conducted in an interview setting with two examiners each hour.
- The Boards are composed of three stations. Each station lasts 60 minutes, and the examiners will assess your knowledge on all areas of neurosurgery.
- Examiners present clinical vignettes for patient management and problem solving. Case histories are given, including appropriate scans and other visual aids to augment the presentation and development of cases. Candidates explain how they would proceed to evaluate and manage the patients, plan and perform operations, if indicated, and deal with complications.
- Subjects covered are the following
  - Neurosurgery: intracranial and vascular diseases.
  - Neurosurgery: spine.
  - Other: critical care, functional and stereotactic neurosurgery, pain, paediatric and congenital disorders, peripheral nerve and plexus, neurology.
- Grades are given on diagnosis, management and handling of complications.

Royal College of Physicians and Surgeons of Canada

The oral component contains eight stations. Each station is 30 minutes in duration and covers three clinical cases.

- The oral component has a total duration of 3 hours with individual stations devoted to intracranial conditions.
- During the examination, you are examined at six stations with two break stations. The stations are (1) spine, (2) spine and peripheral nerves, (3) cranial (vascular), (4) cranial (trauma), (5) cranial (oncology) and (6) paediatrics.
- The oral component of the examination covers a broad range of clinically applied knowledge and performance, particularly the following:
  - Clinical management skills (including neuroradiological interpretation).
  - Surgical problem solving.
  - Judgement and safety.
  - Communication skills.
  - Health care collaboration and management skills.
- This examination emphasizes diagnostics and immediate management.
- If the examiner asks you multiple questions about a similar topic or repeats the question after you answered it, it is a hint that you should change your answer.
- Avoid erroneous actions that may harm patients because you will be deemed unsafe.
- Listen carefully to your examiner. The examiners try to assist during your examination.
- Have a pen and paper at hand to write down silent features. This avoids the need for you to ask the examiner to repeat questions.

European Association of Neurosurgical Societies

- In 1983, the oral component was established in Ljubljana by a joint effort of EANS/UEMS. The exam has evolved over the years and currently follows the Royal College of Surgeons Examination format.

- The examination runs over a half day per candidate. The examination, in the English language, consists of three parts, each lasting 1 hour. Five to eight cases are discussed per hour.
- The exam is conducted in an interview setting with two examiners, experienced neurosurgeons from a European country.
- During these 3 hours the candidate will, therefore, meet six different European examiners, each of whom will give an independent score.
  - 1st hour is dedicated to operative neurosurgery of brain and skull (cranial).
  - 2nd hour covers operative neurosurgery of spine and cord (spine).
  - 3rd hour will cover topics that have not been adequately covered in the first two hours (open).
- The examination is a clinical problem solving and patient management test.
- Case histories are given, and where appropriate neuroimaging and other visual aids are used to augment the presentation and development of cases.
- If the candidate had a borderline/failure performance (failure is <50%) then he or should would have the opportunity to go to an extra fourth station, where the chief examiner participates as an examiner to determine if the candidate should pass. The two examiners in each station come from different EANS member countries.
- The examination questions are standardized, but there is an opportunity for open questioning.

Overall, there are essential differences and different styles among the three examinations. It is important to rely on the three main fundamentals: **knowledge, skills** and **confidence.** There are two very important skills that are beneficial: **organization** and **examination skills.** There is a difference between a candidate who is well organized compared to a candidate who is randomly providing answers. Candidates with excellent examination skills will also have a clear advantage.

To improve your **knowledge**: read more with a critical eye; **skills**: practise and improve your weak areas; **confidence**: comes with knowledge, experience and practice.

American Board of Neurological Surgery (ABNS)
Royal College of Physicians and Surgeons of Canada (FRCSC)
European Association of Neurosurgical Societies (EANS)

Board exam	Emphasis	Mandatory stations	Penalty station	Station duration per day	Failure rate
American	Diagnosis and complication identification plus management including surgical technique	3	No	60 min	Variable Lower
Canadian	Diagnosis and management including some surgical technique questions	8 (6 exam stations and 2 break stations)	No	30 min	15–20%
European	Emphasis on diagnosis and management, but asks fewer surgical technique questions	5 (3 exam stations and 2 break stations)	Yes, one station at the end of the day	45 min	35–45%

Royal Australasian College of Surgeons

Independent specialty neurosurgery practice in Australia and New Zealand is dependent on award of the FRACS (Neurosurgery). This is awarded by the Royal College of Surgeons of Australia and New Zealand at the completion of the training programme. The training programme is administered by the Neurosurgical Society of Australasia (NSA) and is based on a specialty-specific version of the Australasian Surgical Education and Training programme (SET). For international medical graduates wishing to apply for FRACS (Neurosurgery), applications are considered on a specific individual basis by the RACS.

Once candidates have been approved for application for the FRACS (Neurosurgery) exam, the exam is held twice a year. To complete the exam, each of the seven components needs to be completed successfully.

The next five clinical/viva components of the exam take place in one centre, and all the candidates are examined over a 3-day period. The exam is split into four short stations lasting 25 minutes each, where the candidate is examined by two examiners ± the chief examiner. Multimedia is used to present visual information, and the examiners question the candidates directly. The four stations consist of anatomy, operative neurosurgery, surgical pathology and neuroradiology. The clinical station takes place within a hospital environment and lasts 50 minutes, with candidates usually reviewing many patients. The clinical examination involves history taking, examination, discussion of findings, management strategy including investigations and operative/non-operative plans. The focus is on safe practice while the candidates demonstrate a depth of knowledge and complex decision making skills appropriate for a qualified competent neurosurgeon. A component of this examination also relates to patient experience and interaction, and candidates are expected to maintain professional standards. Following the clinical examination, the examiners convene to discuss the candidates and their outcome. When the decisions have been made, candidates from all specialties gather and are given their results. Successful candidates are then invited to join their examiners for a celebration ceremony.

Overall preparation is variable among candidates, but most surgeons will study for approximately a year before the exam. Aim to cover a comprehensive list of topics based on a variety of sources. Approximately 3 months before the exam, candidates should focus on past papers. There are past written papers available from the Neurosurgical Society of Australasia dating back approximately 10 years (a total of 40 papers). Practise performing these examinations under exam conditions and ask senior consultants for feedback. The written exam requires practice. Your time allocation is critical, so adhering to time limits under exam conditions prepares you for the real examination. The written exam is a combination of topics and short and long answers, but several topics have recurred over the years. The following table lists these recurrent topics in order of frequency of appearance in the exams. This can also be used as a topic preparation list.

The vivas are more difficult to prepare for, but ask previously successful candidates and senior consultants to help you prepare by quizzing you on anatomy and operative surgery. Neuroradiologists will invariably have selections of neuroradiology teaching slides, and there are several books to help radiology trainees prepare for their final fellowship exams, which can be used as preparation tools for the neurological sections.

The histopathology viva is a challenge. The WHO book on histopathology classification is an invaluable tool, and all the tumours in this book should be recognizable together with understanding of special stains and criteria for classification of the different tumour grades. Your local neuropathologist may be helpful in showing you historical slides and asking you to describe the salient features. In the viva, the histology slides are accompanied by a radiology image, which helps to guide the pathological diagnosis. The examiners want candidates to describe the relevant histopathological features visible.

The clinical exam is critical to prepare for, and examiners are looking for a polished comprehensive examination and the ability to pick up a variety of simple and complex signs and to put the patient at ease. After examination, further investigations and management strategy are discussed. There are usually combinations of quick cases (e.g. spot diagnoses) such as peripheral nerve wasting patterns or neurophakomatosis, together with more comprehensive cases. It is imperative that you practise examining patients because you must not be thinking about what to test for next but rather focussing on identifying the clinical signs and putting them together. Common clinical cases will involve cranial nerve, brachial plexus and peripheral nerve pathology. Other common cases include syringomyelia, myelopathy, spinal cord injury syndromes and radiculopathies. Examiners will expect candidates to identify the signs and tailor the examination to obtaining a diagnosis while making sure that the specific requests of the examiners are completed.

Clinical anatomy and embryology

- Neuroanatomy of bladder control (2003, 2005)
- Anterior cerebral artery (2010)
- Anterior choroidal artery (2009)
- Blood–brain barrier (2005, 2007)
- L4/5 anatomy (2007, 2010)
- Conduction aphasia (2000)
- Foot drop (2003, 2007, 2010)
- Hypothalamus (2007)
- Internal capsule (1998)
- Internal carotid artery (2011)
- Stupor and coma (1997, 2009)
- Third ventricle (2006)
- Vertebral artery (2008)
- Wallenberg's syndrome (2005)
- Development of cerebellum (2003, 2006)
- Development of neural crest (1994)
- Development of spinal cord (2005)

Peripheral nerves

- Autonomic nervous system – upper limbs (1991, 1994, 2001)
- Ulnar nerve (1998, 2004, 2005, 2008, 2011)
- Brachial plexus (2003, 2007)
- Carpal tunnel syndrome (2001)
- Common peroneal nerve (2000, 2008)
- Foot drop (2003, 2007, 2010)
- Thoracic outlet syndrome (2005, 2008)
- Meralgia paraesthetica (1992, 2006)
- Motor neuron disease (2001)
- Repair of peripheral nerves (1998)
- Sciatic nerve (1999)
- Suprascapular nerve (2002)

Epilepsy, pain and functional

- Perioperative epilepsy (1990, 1995, 1996)
- Temporal lobe epilepsy (2002, 2008, 2011)
- Status epilepticus (2007)
- Surgery for epilepsy (2003)
- Hippocampal sclerosis (1997, 2001)
- Trigeminal neuralgia (1996, 1998 twice, 2001, 2004, 2006, 2008, 2011)
- Anaesthesia dolorosa (2004)
- Glossopharyngeal neuralgia (2002, 2006)
- Hemifacial spasm (2005)
- Parkinson's disease (2004)
- Spinal cord stimulation (2005)

Paediatrics

- Anterior sacral meningocele (2005)
- Arachnoid cyst (1996)
- Cerebellar mutism (2000)
- Chiari malformation (2002, 2004, 2006, 2007)
- Craniosynostosis (1991, 1995, 1996, 2002, 2004, 2006, 2010)
- Dandy Walker syndrome (1999)
- Depressed skull fractures in the newborn (1992,1996)
- Diastomatomyelia (1995, 2009)
- Epilepsy in childhood (2009)
- Growing fractures (1992, 1995, 2000)
- Hydrocephalus in children (1993, 2000)
- IVH in premature newborn (2011)
- Lipomyelomeningocele (1999, 2004)
- Medulloblastoma (2007)
- Non-accidental injury (2009)
- Paediatrics trauma (1999)
- Tethered cord syndrome (1997, 2003, 2011)

Infection

- Brain abscess (1995, 1996, 1999, 2000, 2004)
- Disc space infection (1996, 1998, 2001, 2005, 2006, 2011)
- Postoperative infection (2006, 2008)
- HIV infection (1991, 2004, 2006)
- Spinal abscess (2005, 2009)

- Subdural empyema (1995,1999)
- Prion disease (2003, 2007)
- Cryptococcal infection (2011)
- Histiocytosis X (1994)
- Intracranial toruloma (2003)
- Prophylactic antibiotics in neurosurgery (1995)

Vascular and radiosurgery

- Intracranial aneurysm (1996, 1999, 2002, 2003, 2004, 2006, 2007)
- Vasospasm (1998, 1999, 2001, 2003, 2007, 2010, 2011)
- Subarachnoid haemorrhage (2000 twice, 2005)
- Cavernous malformation (1996, 2001, 2007)
- AVM – cerebral (2000, 2004, 2009)
- AVM – spinal (1996, 2001)
- Carotid endarterectomy (1993, 2005)
- Clinical grading of SAH (2000, 2005)
- Dural arteriovenous fistula (2002)
- MCA stroke management (2009)
- Moya-Moya disease (2005)
- Mycotic intracranial aneurysm (1991, 1999)
- Neuroprotection during vascular surgery (2009)
- Stereotactic radiosurgery (1999, 2001)
- Vertebral artery dissection (2006)

Trauma

- Carotid artery injury/dissection (1992, 1999, 2001)
- Extradural haemorrhage (1990, 1991, 1996, 1997)
- Diffuse axonal injury (1995, 1996, 1999)
- Head injury – outcome prediction (1998, 2004, 2008)
- Head injury – mannitol (1994, 1999, 2001)
- Subdural haemorrhage – chronic (1998, 2001, 2010)
- Trauma management (2000 twice)
- Traumatic CSF fistula (1991, 2000, 2006)
- Brain oedema (2000)
- Burst fracture (2001)
- Cerebral blood flow (2000)
- Gunshot wounds (2004)
- Head injury – ICP (2002, 2010, 2011)

- Head injury – imaging (2001, 2009)
- Head injury – seizure prophylaxis (2010)
- Penetrating brain injury (2000)
- Subdural haemorrhage – acute (2005, 2011)
- Skull fractures (1998)
- Thoracolumbar fractures (2011) Spine

Spine

- Syringomyelia (1991, 1999, 2000, 2001, 2005, 2008)
- Lumbar spondylolisthesis (1992, 1999, 2005, 2006, 2009)
- Cervical disc prolapse (2000, 2003, 2010 twice, 2011)
- Cervical myelopathy (1997, 2000, 2004, 2005)
- Lumbar disc prolapse (1995, 2000, 2004)
- Cervical facet dislocation (1994, 2010)
- C2 fractures (1999, 2004, 2008)
- Atlanto-axial instability (2006, 2009)
- C1 fractures (2001)
- Ankylosing spondylitis (1996)
- Lumbar fusion surgery (2007)
- Monitoring during spinal surgery (2001)
- Spinal tumour (2000, 2003 twice, 2009)
- Thoracic disc prolapse (2007, 2008)

Tumours

- Meningiomas – all areas
- Pituitary adenoma (1997, 1999, 2003, 2004, 2006, 2009)
- Pituitary apoplexy (2000, 2001, 2006, 2007, 2009, 2010)
- Acromegaly (1990, 1996, 2004)
- Cushing's disease (2003, 2005)
- Empty sella syndrome (2008)
- Hypophysitis (2009)
- Acoustic neuroma (1994, 2001, 2004, 2006)
- Brainstem glioma (1999, 2005)
- Cavernous sinus tumour (1999)
- Central neurocytoma (1999, 2000, 2002, 2003)
- Cerebral lymphoma (1996, 1999)
- Chemotherapy for cerebral glioma (2001, 2005)
- Chordoma (1994)
- Classification of brain tumours (2003)

- Colloid cysts (2007, 2009)
- Cortical dysplasia (2005)
- Craniopharyngioma (2003, 2008)
- Dysembryoplastic neuroepithelial tumours (1994, 2006, 2010)
- Ganglioglioma (1994)
- Glioblastoma multiforme (2004, 2011)
- Germinoma (2004)
- Glomus jugulare tumours (2001)
- Metastasis (1991)
- Oligodendroglioma (2000, 2001, 2004, 2005, 2009)
- Pilocytic astrocytoma (1999
- Pineal region tumour (1991, 2005, 2006, 2010)
- Trigeminal schwannoma (2010)
- Neurofibromatosis type 1 (2001)
- Neurofibromatosis type 2 (1995, 2000, 2003, 2009)
- von Hippel-Lindau syndrome (1999)

Miscellaneous

- Air and fat embolism (1992, 1998)
- Aspirin and neurosurgery (1993, 1994)
- Brain death (1995, 2003, 2006)
- Cerebral blood flow (2009)
- Disseminated intravascular coagulopathy (1998)
- Driving postcraniotomy (1998, 2004)
- Endoscopy (2005)
- Evolving hemispheric mass lesion (2010)
- Glasgow Outcome Scale (2003)
- Heparin-induced thrombocytopenia (2007)
- House-Brackman grading scale (1999, 2001, 2003, 2004, 2009, 2010)
- Hyponatremia (2006, 2008, 2010)
- Hypothermia (1992, 1994, 2005)
- Immuno-histochemistry (1994)
- Informed consent (1994, 2001, 2004)
- Neurosurgical audits (2007)
- Osteoplastic versus free bone flaps (2000)
- Peptic ulcer prophylaxis (1998)
- Atlanto-axial instability (2006, 2009)
- Physiology of clotting (2004)
- Postoperative analgesia (2001)
- Preoperative embolisation (2007)
- Thromboprophylaxis in neurosurgery (2010)
- Intracerebral haemorrhage (1997, 2003, 2010)
- Functional MRI (2003)
- MRI (1993)
- Neuronavigation (2002)
- Transcranial Doppler (1998)

Conclusion

Preparing for the neurosurgical examination is a challenge. Your revision must not be rushed. This book serves as a guide with which you can test yourself on examination-style questions and obtain the correct answers. This book covers all clinical sections of the examination in a comprehensive and structured manner. Organize your revision in a productive way in order to address the various conditions that will be encountered. This book serves as a guide and a revision aid, but it cannot replace examining patients with clinical signs in hospitals and outpatient settings. By acquiring the essential knowledge and skills and through independent study during your training, you will be able to communicate your knowledge to the examiners.

Assemble your 'tool box'

- Caliper.
- Coin (e.g. 50 pence piece or a quarter).
- Cotton wool balls.
- Key.
- Medical hat pins (red and white).
- Neurotips.
- Paper clip.
- Pen.
- Picture of a famous political figure (e.g. the Queen or the President of the United States).
- Ruler.
- Snellen's pocket eye chart.
- Tendon hammer (e.g. MDF Queen Square Hammer).
- Tongue depressor.
- Torch.
- Tuning forks (c128 Hz and c512 Hz).

Assimilate your knowledge into clinical practise. Practise performing regular neurological examinations to ensure that you have a structured planned routine.

Enjoy the journey!

How to succeed

Viva advice

Preparation for the viva starts when you begin to study for the whole examination. There are two phases – 'early' and 'late'. In this early phase, the emphasis is on acquiring knowledge. The earlier you begin the revision, not only will you be better prepared, the more relaxed you will be during the exam. At this stage, the strategy is to minimize risk by selecting the 'hot topics'. Our advice is to avoid extremes. On the one hand, you should not waste valuable time with in-depth research into highly specialized topics. On the other hand, avoid large gaps in your knowledge by only concentrating on the major topics. Ensure you have a structured revision timetable, organize your thoughts and have a strategy to tackle the exam.

Allocation of time – knowledge sampling

When it comes to the assimilation of knowledge, a simple fact remains – you cannot know everything. The key is to have insight into the topics (either written, knowledge-based clinical technique or viva discussion) of 'high yield' and spend more time on these topics and less on those that are unlikely to be encountered. Developing a system to hone this insight is key, especially when the examination dates loom close and increasing stress levels make this task more haphazard and less efficient.

For the neurosurgical examination, there is a core body of neurosurgical information that is essential, the **must know.** Beyond that there is additional knowledge and wisdom, which can be considered as **should know,** with a third sphere of content, which can be considered as **may know**. The examiner's task is to ensure that the exam candidate demonstrates a robust understanding of 'must know' topics to pass. Assessment of the 'should know' and 'may know' content is directed at determining the depth and breadth of neurosurgical training, which also serves as a surrogate marker to determine a 'rank' of sorts among peers. This provides a structure with which to understand the selection of topics encountered within the objective assessment criteria of the multiple choice questions (MCQs), standards based assessment (SBA), clinical and viva answers.

Within the entire neurosurgical curriculum there is of course a sub-division of topics. Taking the example of paediatric neurosurgery, the curriculum is going to encompass a number of topics, as illustrated in this 'knowledge cloud' (see Figure 1.1). Within this illustrative selection, the topics in larger font will be generally considered 'must know', with the smaller fonts successively representing 'should know' and 'may know' domains. Considering the time limitations of the examinations, the exam can only 'sample' a section of this knowledge cloud with some MCQs, viva questions or clinical cases based on the topic chosen. The probability of an individual topic being selected for questioning is directly proportional to the importance of the topic as perceived by the examiner. Thus the probability likelihood of 'must know' questions is greater than 'should know' topics, which is greater than 'may know' questions.

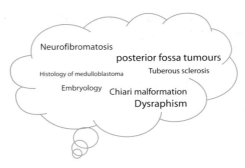

Figure 1.1 Example of 'knowledge cloud' of paediatric neurosurgery topics

These principles are commonly understood but often not considered either early on or very late in exam revision. When beginning the bulk of exam preparation, the key is to elucidate the 'probability algorithms' in the minds of the examiners, which are very well replicated if one were to *discuss the subspecialty with senior neurosurgeons* in your unit. For example, a paediatric neurosurgical consultant with several years of experience will be able to prioritize the 'must know/should know/may know' topics in paediatrics. This information is what needs to be understood to allocate exam preparation time to the topics, not the list of conditions listed in a neurosurgical exam preparation textbook.

With respect to the final stages of preparing for the exam, it is this prioritization that should determine the allocation of time needed to cover all topics. For example, on the evening before the exams, you should confirm that you have rehearsed your answers on the key topics. It would be a better use of time to spend a few minutes perfecting the delivery of answers for such a topic rather than opening up a histopathology book to review the detailed findings of paraffin sections for a specific tumour. Though clearly the latter can be asked, an inability to answer the question will not fail a candidate. But a less polished, hesitant answer about the common differentials of brain tumours that requires prompting by the examiner can risk your performing below the accepted standard.

In essence one needs to consider that only a small percentage of the entire curriculum is going to be sampled and, by definition, one cannot know everything that can be asked. So it is important to bolster knowledge and delivery of answers for the more likely sampled topics rather than to devote equal time to all topics.

Late phase preparation

There is often a significant period of time between completion of the written component of the examination and commencement of the oral and clinical sections. This is an important 'late' phase of preparation. Factual knowledge has already been assessed in the written component, and the viva is meant to explore your logical understanding of this assimilated information. *During this later stage of viva revision, prepare the expected answer and do not attempt to acquire new knowledge* (hence the importance of the 'early' phase of preparation). The experience of most candidates who have taken the oral and clinical components is that they overwhelmingly relied on their previous experience and knowledge, rather than new information that they acquired during the 'late' phase of their preparation. Under stressful conditions, problem-solving skill defaults to past experience and pattern recognition. Managing performance during these stressful conditions is the key to success, and much can be gained by understanding how we perform within these scenarios, as detailed later.

There are numerous examples. During the operative viva, there will be questions directed to how to avoid and address intra-operative complications, and, during the Long Case, what investigations are required to help obtain the underlying diagnosis. This strategy returns back to your preparation in the early phase. In addition to acquiring knowledge, you should be in the correct frame of mind in preparing for this exam in your daily practice. Take note while on the wards, in the outpatient setting and in the operating room. Last minute cramming is less likely to be rewarding. Finally, no matter how well prepared you are for the exam, it is most difficult to answer a question that you have not prepared in advance. It is advised during your late preparation to select possible topics (surprisingly, these turn out to be fewer than you would have thought), imagine the various possible questions (putting yourself in the examiner's position) and prepare your final answers.

The skill of answering viva questions

A very useful concept to understand performance in the examinations is the Dreyfus model[1] of adult skill acquisition. After all the examination is a platform to demonstrate your 'performance' and thus it can be vastly improved by studying the

Table 1.1 Dreyfus model of skill acquisition[1]

Level	Description	Analogy
Novice	• Rigid adherence to taught rules or plans • Little situational perception • No discretionary judgement	New learner driver who needs to be told the exact rules of driving, e.g. change gear from 1 to 2 when speed is greater than 10 mph, look at left and rear mirror when turning left etc.
Advanced beginner	• Guidelines for action based on attributes or aspects (aspects are global characteristics of situations recognizable only after some prior experience) • Situational perception still limited • All attributes and aspects are treated separately and given equal importance	With experience the 'advanced beginner' driver starts to notice the sound of the engine (high revs) as a cue to going up through the gears. . . learns more cues or rules that determine driving, e.g. how close is the car in front (if too close need to go slower) and how close is the cyclist on the side, etc.
Competent	• Coping with crowdedness • Now sees actions at least partially in terms of longer-term goals • Conscious deliberate planning • Standardized and routinized procedures	Driver starts to learn to 'ignore rules' as can't actively think about too many rules but starts to simply know intuitively how fast to go, which gear to take. . . e.g. when late can start to make changes to drive faster etc.
Proficient	• Sees situations holistically rather than in terms of aspects • Sees what is most important in a situation • Perceives deviations from the normal pattern • Decision-making less laboured • Uses maxims for guidance, whose meaning varies according to the situation	Driver goes into a turn with relatively high speed and just realizes that the car seems to be going too fast. . . considers options of taking foot off accelerator pedals or breaking. . . decides to gently depress break. . . car achieves speed which driver is more comfortable with.
Expert	• No longer relies on rules, guidelines or maxims • Intuitive grasp of situations based on deep tacit understanding • Analytic approaches used only in novel situations, when problems occur • Vision of what is possible	High-speed turn on wet road on motorway. . . an 'expert' driver will intuitively take foot gently off accelerator to allow car to achieve and maintain optimal speed. . . all this can be happening while carrying on a conversation uninterrupted with passengers. . . all actions are automatic.

stepwise improvement inherent in any complex adult skill acquisition. The concept is perhaps best understood by considering the analogy of driving (see Table 1.1). The performance varies as tabulated from a novice who has to be told the exact rules of driving (when to exactly change gears etc.) to an expert driver who can chauffeur a car at high speeds at night in wet conditions without the passengers becoming uncomfortable on the turns.

Similarly in a viva exam situation, the ability to present can range from a novice to an expert. The 'novice' will be thinking of the 'rules' of answering and trying to use them to formulate the answers. For example, when asked about a scan showing a left sylvian fissure subarachnoid haemorrhage (SAH), he or she will think, 'What is this? Is it a traumatic or spontaneous SAH? Should I use the WFNS or Fisher grade to describe it? What are the other things I should think of?'

An 'expert', on the other hand, may say, 'This 50-year-old old female has a history typical of SAH and the scan confirms a Fisher grade 3, WFNS grade 1 spontaneous SAH with early hydrocephalus. I would bring the patient across urgently for a computed tomography (CT) angiogram to investigate for a middle cerebral artery (MCA) aneurysm'.

The 'expert' is one who has become so experienced with dealing with a situation, presenting it before seniors and treating similar patients that the description of the scan and management plan comes automatically, and he or she does not have to think about what to say. The comforting view is that most candidates who attempt postgraduate exams will be at least at the 'competent' level or higher in dealing with most common cases. They therefore need to manage their stress level just enough to allow their level of 'skill acquisition' to show through in the discussions they have with the examiners.

Managing stress

The Yerkes–Dodson Law (Figure 1.2),[3] or the stress/performance curve, is a well-studied topic in various human endeavours. At its essence this law merely states that initially performance improves with increasing levels of 'stress' or 'arousal'. However, beyond a certain point, further increases in stress result in worsening performance and are counterproductive. Though this principle was first scientifically demonstrated by Yerkes–Dodson in animal biological models over a century ago, it is grounded in common sense and has been shown to be appropriate for human biological responses as well.[4] What is important to realize is that the relationship between performance and stress is dependent on the complexity of the task being performed.

A natural corollary of this fact is that in a very stressful situation, such as a post-graduate examination, candidates will continue to perform well at a task that is 'easy' for them. (They will follow the curve to the right of the diagram.) During the same exam setting they will invariably end up worse at tasks that are 'complex' for them (curve to the left). So if they were already 'proficient' (stage 4 of the Dreyfus model detailed earlier) at performing a fundoscopy examination, despite supra-normal stress levels they may still continue to perform as if 'competent' at the examination and thus easily meet the criteria the examiners are looking for to pass a candidate. But a candidate who was 'competent' may drop down to the 'advanced beginner' stage and then find himself or herself in trouble in regard to meeting the minimum requirements expected.

It is therefore imperative that candidates do not modify significantly their examination techniques close to the examinations. Such changes to the subtle sequence of steps required to perform even a relatively simple task, without significant prior practice, will mean candidates will be more likely to behave as if the task is a 'complex' one, with risk of poorer performance at high stress levels.

Performance in a postgraduate exam is just that – a performance. It involves a plethora of 'soft' skills, which complement the presentation of knowledge and application of the core medical subject being examined. These need to be presented at 'competent' level or better and include the following:

- verbal fluency;
- syntax emphasis;
- eye contact;
- body language;
- confidence (a combination of the above).

Most candidates are stressed over the ability to present an adequate amount of content to the examiner, but it is more important to present

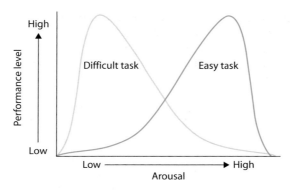

Figure 1.2 Yerkes-Dodson Law.

whatever content they know in a systematic and balanced approach and in a manner that fits the 'profile' that the examiner seeks to confirm. In most UK postgraduate/Royal College fellowship examinations, this is the 'profile' of a first day consultant in the relevant specialty.

An illustration may be the classic example of a discussion of pancreatitis. Many undergraduate books list mnemonics of the causes and interestingly many trainees seem to retain 'scorpion bite' as one of the causes. In a membership exam, one may inadvertently recite this as one of the causes and follow this with the more common causes, such as alcoholism and gallstones, and pass the exam. However in a postgraduate exam, the examiner (who almost certainly would be a practising consultant) would not take kindly to such a clinically insignificant cause of pancreatitis in the western world being volunteered as the initial answer. He or she would be seeking to hear a clinically experienced discussion wherein the candidate may start with stating that alcoholism and gallstones are the most common pathologies. Then perhaps they might expect the candidate to temper his or her suspicions – perhaps more to gallstones if the patient was a middle-aged woman and more to alcoholism if the demographics were significantly different, favouring it as a potential cause. Further detailed discussions may end up with the probability of different pathologies causing pancreatitis (even perhaps scorpion bite), its mechanism, treatment and even recent publications on the subject. Key here is the chronology of the discussion, which represents the expected 'pattern' of behaviour and

answers from a first day consultant. A candidate would almost certainly pass not even having mentioned a scorpion bite!

Taking advantage

Understanding the exam pattern and psychology of the examiners is the best aid a candidate can have for better performance. Knowing the basic facts is important. Usually, the viva will start with simple topics and then the questions will have a crescendo of increasing complexity. Therefore, it is not advised to start with a complex answer because this could be pretentious and counterproductive; similarly if you fail to adequately answer the remaining complex questions, this should not affect your overall performance.

Provided it is not at the very beginning of the session, if you are asked about a topic that you are well prepared for, take advantage of this. You can guide the examiner through your answer to demonstrate your thorough knowledge. Here the aim should be to obtain the 'gold medal' in these situations. Demonstrate that you are a safe surgeon with a solid foundation in the basic topics. Most important, be attentive and listen to the examiners. They may provide hints and point you in the correct direction. Most candidates under estimate the willingness of the examiners to help during the examination. With the vast majority of examiners, it is not a confrontation or an exercise in psychological warfare. This begins by the questions being asked and dictates how long and comprehensive your answer should be. The best strategy is to 'define, classify and then amplify'.

For example, if asked about methods of evaluating cerebral blood flow (CBF), define, classify (invasive vs. non-invasive or quantitative vs. qualitative) and then amplify (mention the various investigations). However, if asked about the application of positron emission tomography (PET) scans in estimation of CBF, concentrate on the details of this specific investigation. Similarly, during the clinical examination, if the examiner directs you towards examining a particular area, then take the hint, and concentrate on this specific area to detect the abnormality. Moreover, the examiner will prompt you to move forward if you are taking too much time in irrelevant areas, or he or she may not interrupt you if the examination is relevant to diagnosing the underlying pathology. If the examiner repeats the question, it is likely that your answer is not appropriate.

Common pitfalls

There are three main reasons why candidates run into difficulties during the oral and clinical examination.

1. Poor presentation of answers

Although the topics and initial questions are standardized, the subsequent questions are based on your previous answers. With a degree of certainty, you can prepare for possible questions that will be asked on a given topic. Complex answers will generate subsequent difficult questions. If you do not know the answer, within reason, tell the examiner that you 'do not know' so you may move on to the next topic.

2. Lack of safe management

Before embarking on any complex management plan, it is important to demonstrate that you have considered all forms of treatment (e.g. conservative, medical and surgical).

3. Misinterpretation of the evidence and non-malleable thinking

Ensure that you read the quoted literature for multiple sources. For example, stating that the International Subarachnoid Aneurysm Trial (ISAT) indicates that endovascular coiling is preferred to aneurysm clipping is correct. But in fact, the literature's findings relate to small (<10 mm) anterior circulation aneurysms. It is best to avoid the terms 'always' and 'never'. The examiner will set to prove you wrong. Moreover, this may represent non-malleable thinking. For example, the statement, 'I "always" use a lumbar drain in aneurysm surgery' will be followed by the examiner providing you with a scan of an MCA aneurysm with a large haematoma, contraindicating the lumbar puncture. Similarly, providing exact figures or percentages should be avoided. This represents knowledge from limited sources.

REFERENCES

1. Dreyfus S, Dreyfus H. A five stage model of the mental activities involved in directed skill acquisition. Operations Research Center, University of Berkeley, 1980.
2. Eraut M. Non-formal learning and tacit knowledge in professional work. *Br J Educ Psychol* 2000; 70(1): 113–136.
3. Yerkes RM, Dodson JD. The relation of strength of stimulus to rapidity of habit-formation. *J Comp Neurol Psychol* 1908; 18: 459–482.
4. Sjöberg H. Interaction of task difficulty, activation, and workload. *J Human Stress* 1977; 3(1): 33–38.

How to plan for specific scenarios

Throughout the oral and clinical neurosurgical examination, you will be provided with different scenarios for management. You must **listen** to the examiner and understand the question being asked. There are endless pitfalls. The following are important examples.

The examiner provided you with a long scenario on a polytrauma case. During the description, you are informed that the patient is localizing to pain, making few incomprehensible sounds and not eye opening to pain. One pupil is noted to be fixed and dilated. It is best not to start your answer by reporting that you will first assess the patient's Glasgow Coma Scale (GCS) and pupils to assess if the patient is in deep coma because this information has already been provided. Similarly, if you are provided with a case in which the patient, a teacher, is suffering from intractable epilepsy despite medical optimization and is being considered for surgery, it is best not to report that based on the patient's occupation and IQ you may or may not propose surgery because this information and decision has already been made.

The following are common scenarios and practical advice on how to answer these 'hot topics'.

Neurovascular scenarios

Sylvian ICH – ruptured MCA aneurysm

Safety – predict variations – specific precautions

If there are no further details about the given scenario, then begin by mentioning the key factors that determine the management of a ruptured aneurysm. The key factors include GCS, rate of deterioration, age, size of haematoma and evidence of mass effect. In patients with low GCS who rapidly deteriorated and harbour a large intracranial haematoma (ICH), then the priority is to treat the increased intracranial pressure (ICP) by medical optimization (e.g. administration of mannitol) followed by craniotomy to evacuate the haematoma and clip the aneurysm. Your answer should be tailored to the specific scenario and demonstrate your safe approach, avoidance of complications, surgical anatomical knowledge and experience. Preoperative planning should include an understanding of the haematoma (location) and the aneurysm (size and projection of the fundus). Planning the head position on the operation table with the size of the craniotomy flap should allow for adequate ICH decompression and the ability to obtain safe proximal control. When evacuating the ICH, be safe and adequate and prevent aneurysm re-rupture. Depending on the anatomical location of the clot, evacuation can be achieved by splitting the distal sylvian fissure away from the expected aneurysm to allow for a trans-sylvian evacuation. In cases of large dominant hemisphere temporal clots, a trans-superior temporal gyrus approach with an anterior corticotomy may be more appropriate. In either case, the initial evacuation should be partial so as not to disturb the tamponade effect of the clot on the underlying aneurysm, but large enough to allow for brain relaxation and access to the basal cisterns for proximal control. Once the aneurysm is clipped, the residual ICH can be evacuated.

If the aneurysm size and configuration are favourable, demonstrate your anatomical knowledge and safety by describing how you would clip the aneurysm. This could include proximal control, dissection of M1, use of temporary clips (preferably distal to the lenticulostriate branch), identification of all M2 branches (look carefully for extra branches – trifurcation rather than bifurcation), circumferential fundus dissection, and assurance that the clip does not occlude or kink any associated branches. The use of intraoperative indocyanine green (ICG) is helpful in these situations.

If you choose to evacuate the ICH and then proceed to endovascular coiling, mention the key safety steps to prevent intraoperative rupture. Following endovascular coiling, be prepared to advise on the potential benefits and complications of periprocedural heparin and antiplatelet agents.

If faced with a ruptured giant aneurysm, a safe option is to perform a decompressive craniectomy. Once the patient has been stabilized, an experienced vascular neurosurgeon can take over the patient's care. If you report preservation of the superficial temporal artery while performing the craniotomy, then proceeding to partial ICH evacuation to allow for brain relaxation, gaining proximal control, dissecting the aneurysm neck, preserving all M2 branches and proceeding to bypass is not the ideal answer. Giant aneurysms should be referred to an experienced vascular surgeon in a multidisciplinary setting, and not addressed by a junior neurosurgeon.

In stable patients, a further option is to select endovascular coiling of the aneurysm followed by evacuation of the ICH, as needed. Demonstrate awareness regarding the use of anticoagulants during the procedure and their reversal prior to craniotomy.

Scenario 1: 28-year-old pregnant woman presents with WFNS Grade I subarachnoid haemorrhage (SAH) from a ruptured 7 mm internal carotid bifurcation aneurysm

Awareness of variations – safety

The key to this scenario is to focus on the management of the SAH and consider the influence of the pregnancy on the recommended treatments.

The management options (conservative, medical, endovascular and surgical) depend on patient selection and the underlying aneurysm. During the first trimester, there is a potential high risk of teratogenic effects of medication and anaesthesia on the fetus. At term, consideration for an elective caesarean section followed by surgery may be the best treatment. There is no standard answer, because each patient is different. If endovascular treatment is chosen, be specific in mentioning shielding the fetus from radiation, positioning the patient (tilting the abdomen to the left side to decrease the compression of the inferior vena cava) and involving the obstetricians.

Scenario 2: 65-year-old man presents with perimesencephalic SAH. The computed tomography angiography (CTA) scan does not demonstrate a vascular abnormality

Awareness of controversy – principles of management

The definition of what constitutes perimesencephalic SAH is debatable. Digital subtraction angiography (DSA) remains the gold standard in diagnosing aneurysms.

Be prepared for debate. Acknowledge the possible diagnostic challenges. Most surgeons would recommend DSA. In the context of perimesencephalic SAH with a negative initial DSA, this would not require further investigations. In practice, the management can be complex. For example, if the patient has evidence of interhemispheric extension (which by definition is minor and still classifies the bleed as a perimesencephalic type), the decision whether or not to repeat an angiography to exclude anterior communicating aneurysm is not clear.

Scenario 3: Counselling a 32-year-old teacher who is diagnosed with an incidental 14 mm anterior communicating aneurysm (ACoA)

Comprehensive – only relevant figures – very specific treatment risks

The counselling includes three discussions: (1) the natural history of the vascular lesion; (2) treatment options with the associated benefits and complications; (3) the psychological impact on the patient. There are two parts to consultation: information giving (explaining the diagnosis) and information gathering (exploring the patient's views and specific worries).

When discussing the natural history of this condition, mention the risk of rupture based on the International Study of Unruptured Intracranial Aneurysms (ISUIA) in reference to size of an anterior circulation aneurysm (see table below).

Mention that you are aware of the limitations of the study, and that the life-long risks still need to be calculated.

Be specific in explaining the risks of treatment that apply particularly to the ACoA aneurysm. Discuss the positive morphological factors for the aneurysm in obtaining a long-term obliteration rate.

Size of aneurysm	Anterior circulation % of rupture rates	Posterior circulation % of rupture rates
< 7 mm	0	2.5
7–12 mm	2.6	14.5
13–24 mm	14.5	18.4
≥25 mm	40	50

Scenario 4: 43-year-old man has recovered well following SAH. He underwent endovascular coiling of a posterior communicating artery (PCoA) aneurysm with a fetal PCoA. At 6 months, his MRI/MRA scan demonstrated a recurrence and partial filling of the aneurysm neck

Awareness of controversy – specific precautions

Demonstrate knowledge regarding the incidence of recurrence, factors that increase recurrence rates (e.g. neck configuration, partial thrombosis, end result at the time of the procedure, smoking) and the special consideration for age and interval to recurrence. Safety is a major component in this clinical examination. Before embarking on treatment options, assess the natural history of the condition. Discuss the different patterns of recurrence, filling of the fundus and, more importantly, the known re-bleeding risk from the recurrent or residual neck. If you decide to quote figures from the literature be aware that there are wide variations in different series.

If re-coiling of the aneurysm is your chosen option then ensure that you demonstrate the possible complications, including the need for stent-assisted recoiling and the importance of not occluding the dominant PCoA. The role of surgical clipping should also be considered. This may be suitable in cases where there is coil impaction. This would allow for application of the aneurysmal clip without retrieval of the coils and preserving the PCoA. Clipping, although technically challenging, would have a better long-term outcome.

Scenario 5: 16-year-old boy presents with controlled seizures and has been diagnosed with a deep insular 2 cm AVM

Safety – defend treatment option – specific results

The key to the questions is that the patient is young with a deep-seated vascular lesion. The life-long risk of bleeding from this AVM should be discussed. The primary aim of treatment is to curtail this risk of bleeding rather than to obtain seizure control. A Randomized Trial of Unruptured Brain Arteriovenous Malformations (ARUBA) interim analysis demonstrated that medical management is superior to intervention in patients with unruptured AVMs. Be safe: surgery for deep-seated AVMs has serious potential risks. Stereotactic radiosurgery can be considered in cases of small AVMs.

Scenario 6: 18-year-old woman, who underwent childhood cranial radiation for leukaemia, presents with sudden onset of upper limb clumsiness, a sensory deficit in the lower face and diplopia. The MRI scan demonstrates a pontine cavernoma with a minor haemorrhage

Knowledge – management options – safety

Consider the young age of this patient in context of the natural history of brainstem cavernomas. Moreover, because the patient has undergone previous whole brain radiation, stereotactic radiation may not be recommended.

Focus on safety. Surgery may not be recommended until a further episode of haemorrhage to allow for a gliotic plane to develop. Mention the specific factors, including location within the pons and the characteristics of the haemorrhage (e.g. whether the bleed presents to the cortical surface or is surrounded by functional neural tissue). Without prompting by the examiner, mention that any associated developmental venous anomaly (DVA) should remain untouched.

Demonstrate your neuroanatomical knowledge by indicating the safe surgical approaches and illustrate position of the various nuclei and tracts in the floor of the fourth ventricle as shown in Figure 2.1.

Tumour scenarios

Scenario 7: 52-year-old man presents with a typical history of migraines. His MRI scan demonstrates a 12 mm colloid cyst with no associated hydrocephalus

Knowledge – specific advice to patient – specific approach

Demonstrate your knowledge regarding the overall management of incidental colloid cysts. This should include the accepted recommendation for treatment if the colloid cyst is symptomatic, >10 mm in size, and located high in the septum pellucidum or in the roof of the third ventricle. Sudden death due to a colloid cyst is rare but an important consideration. Discuss the significance of the presence or absence of hydrocephalus in

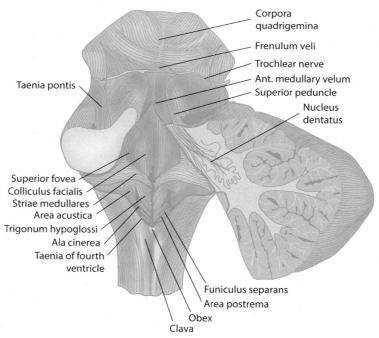

Figure 2.1 Anatomy of the fourth ventricle (see Scenario 7).

selecting a surgical approach. Safety is the major key issue; do not underestimate the morbidity (including memory impairment) and mortality following transcallosal surgery.

In this case, take into consideration of the history of migraines, which would be problematic if a conservative approach is adopted. Also advise the patient to seek urgent medical attention if symptoms progress.

Scenario 8: 43-year-old woman diagnosed with a left-sided low-grade glioma in the opercular part of the inferior frontal gyrus

Knowledge of natural history and possible role of adjuvant treatment – safety – intraoperative plan

The purpose of this scenario is to discuss the natural history, prognosis, role of intraoperative monitoring given its anatomical location, extent of surgical resection and role of adjuvant treatment. Start your answer by covering the basics well. Be safe and not a master surgeon. Then you can move into a discussion regarding the role of intraoperative neurophysiological monitoring and white matter tract stimulation for speech versus the benefits and limitations of intraoperative MRI. If you are not fully aware of the adjuvant therapy trials, inform the examiner that you do not know rather than providing inaccurate figures and conclusions.

Scenario 9: 56-year-old man presents with a recurrence in his high-grade glioma. Consider his further treatment options

Case-specific decision-making – knowledge of adjuvant therapies

Explain the clear indications for further treatment. Explain your reasoning when considering the various factors in your decision-making process. These factors include age, performance status, interval to recurrence, response to previous treatment, patient's expectations, availability of further adjuvant treatment options, accessibility for further resection, safety of further surgery and prediction of resectability. The first step is to confirm that the lesion is recurrent tumour rather than radionecrosis. The discussion may include the various diagnostic modalities with their sensitivities, specificities and limitations (positron emission tomography [PET], perfusion MRI, etc.). For a patient undergoing further surgery, the use of Gliadel wafers (prolifeprosan 20 with carmustine implant) should be considered. Be aware of the benefits, side effects, limitations and contraindications to their use. Discuss the role of glioma biomarkers in classifying and grading gliomas. The overall survival or progression-free survival is longer in patients with O(6)-methylguanine-DNA methyltransferase (MGMT) promoter methylation and *IDH-1* mutations. This is an opportunity to demonstrate current, evidence-based literature.

Epilepsy scenario

Scenario 10: 27-year-old university lecturer presents with three to four uncontrolled seizures per month. His underlying diagnosis is presumed hippocampal sclerosis. Perform an adequate preoperative assessment

Individual considerations – relevant assessment for surgery – understanding investigations

Before answering the question, consider the relevant facts that have been provided. It is best to avoid the obvious pitfall by stating that you will establish the patient's seizure frequency and recommend management according to the patient age and occupation. These are facts that have already been provided. Do not waste valuable time repeating established facts.

Because the question mentions a preoperative assessment, it is fair to say that you would re-confirm the indications for surgery by taking a detailed history, performing a neurological examination and reviewing all investigations. Nevertheless, as a surgeon you should mention that it is important to establish that the seizures are 'true' rather than 'pseudo', understand the semiology of the seizures, ensure that the patient was compliant in taking anticonvulsants, ensure that sufficient time was afforded for medical optimization and determine if overall quality of life has been assessed. The question indicates that the assessment has been performed, but it is important to confirm the diagnosis, localize the target and report on the safety of surgery. The initial workup includes blood tests, a brain MRI scan and electroencephalography (EEG) with video telemetry. This may lead you to discuss the different MRI sequences and hippocampal volume assessment. If there is doubt regarding the localization of the lesion, discuss the role, principles and limitations of ictal and interictal PET, single-photon emission computed tomography (SPECT) and subdural and depth electrodes. In addition, demonstrate an understanding of functional magnetic resonance imaging (fMRI) and the Wada test. The patient's speech, memory and neuropsychological state will also need to be assessed.

3

Long and short cases

History taking

As a reminder, at the end of your history taking and prior to the start of the clinical examination, you should, to a great extent, be able to localize the pathological process, determine the underlying aetiology and establish the urgency for treatment. The actual clinical examination serves to confirm your hypothesis.

Clinical examination

The assessment begins when you take a detailed history from the patient. Assess for cognitive function, speech, posture, surgical scars, facial asymmetry, inattention and ophthalmoplegia. As mentioned above, at the end of the history the localization of the pathological process should be achieved and then you will be able to perform a targeted examination. Your clinical examination serves to confirm the diagnosis and determine the patient's overall management.

It is noteworthy that when you examine limb power it varies depending on whether it is targeted to assess intracranial or spinal function. For cranial cases, the general pattern of the motor weakness is global (e.g. evidence of a pronator drift). For spinal cases, inspect for specific muscle wasting and examine power in myotomal patterns. Avoid examining two movements sharing the same root or myotome value. It is recommended that you ask the patient to perform the movement to be examined and you oppose it rather than the other way round; e.g. for elbow extension, ask the patient to keep their arm straight and tell them to prevent you from flexing it. The reason is to examine a pure movement. If you ask them to straighten the elbow against resistance, there is a chance the patient may use 'trick' movements such as supination to compensate for a subtle extension weakness. As long as you demonstrate competence and identify the neurological deficit, any method you select will be acceptable. If patients can walk or support their whole body weight on their tiptoes and heels, that will make the power in ankle movements MRC Grade 5. Include the assessment of gait and Romberg's test (to assess the dorsal columns of the spinal cord).

During the long and short cases, the candidate should have a systematic approach to obtaining a clinical history, performing the clinical examination, interpreting the appropriate investigations and obtaining the underlying diagnosis. A clear management plan should include conservative, medical and surgical treatments. Discussion regarding the patient's overall prognosis may also be included.

Having a balance is important. A speedy, confident and thorough but targeted examination is recommended. Avoid a cursory and rapid examination because it will appear that you are going through the motions rather than actually examining the patient.

During your preparation, devise a logical and efficient scheme for the examination and be prepared to justify why you examine in a particular way. You will be assessed in the interpretation of the clinical signs and what further investigations are warranted. Formulate a list of possible cases and prepare your targeted answers.

Short cases

- Chiasmal/suprasellar lesions.
- Pituitary dysfunction.
  - Acromegaly.
  - Cushing's disease.
- Speech problems and assessments.
  - Dysphasia.
  - Dysarthria.
  - Dysphonia.
- Short history taking.
  - Facial pain, e.g. trigeminal neuralgia.
  - Headache, e.g. benign intracranial hypertension (BIH).
  - Seizure/syncope.
  - Transient neurologic deficit.
- Higher cortical assessments, e.g. frontal, temporal, parietal and occipital lobes.
- Eyes.
  - Cranial nerve III palsy.
  - Diplopia.
  - Internuclear ophthalmoplegia (INO).
  - Carotico-cavernous fistula.
  - Parinaud's syndrome.
- Limbs.
  - Carpal tunnel syndrome.
  - Hemi-cord syndromes.
  - Brachial nerve palsy – ulnar, median and radial nerve palsies.
  - Myelopathy – cervical or thoracic.
  - Radiculopathy.
  - Numb hands/feet, e.g. peripheral neuropathy.
  - Foot drop.
- Gait.
  - Normal pressure hydrocephalus (NPH).
  - Cerebellar.
- Neurocutaneous syndrome.
  - Tuberous sclerosis.
  - Neurofibromatosis (NF-1, NF-2).
  - Von Hippel–Lindau syndrome.
  - Sturge–Weber syndrome.
  - Osler–Weber Rendu syndrome.
- Functional.
  - Tremors.
  - Parkinson's disease.
- Others.
  - Dural fistulas.

Examples of short cases

Cranial

- Assess this patient's speech.
- Assess this patient's swallowing.
- A patient presents with weakness in his right hand. Examine his frontal and parietal lobe function.
- A patient suffers from facial pain. Take a history and examine the patient.
- A patient suffers from gait imbalance. Perform the relevant examination.
- A patient suffers from headaches. Take brief history and examine the patient.

Eyes

- A patient has blurred vision. Examine his eyes.
- A patient presents with ptosis, miosis and anhidrosis. Examine the patient for Horner's syndrome.
- A patient has a bulging eye. Assess for pulsatile proptosis.

Ears

- A patient suffers from tinnitus. Perform a focused neurological examination.

Endocrine

- A patient reports that he is no longer able to wear his wedding ring and his shoe size has increased. Perform the relevant examination.
- A patient reports weight gain despite careful dietary control. Perform the relevant examination.
- Spot diagnosis of acromegaly and Cushing's syndrome.

Functional

- A patient has a tremor. Perform a focused neurological examination.
- A patient suffers from long-standing seizures. Examine his temporal lobe function.
- A patient suffers from Parkinson's disease. Perform a focused examination.

Paediatrics

- Parents are concerned by their child's increased head size. Examine for craniosynostosis and classify the relevant subtypes.
- A child has been diagnosed with hydrocephalus secondary to a pineal tumour. Examine and investigate this child.

Spine

- A patient has a foot drop. Perform the relevant examination.
- A patient presents with reduced grip strength and dropping objects. Perform the relevant examination.

At the end, you may be asked the following:

- Summarize your findings.
- What is the likely diagnosis?

Define, classify and amplify

- Definition.
- Incidence.
- Aetiology.
- Causes: Use the mnemonic: INVITED MD.
  Infection.
  Neoplasia.
  Vascular.
  Inflammatory/immune.
  Trauma.
  Endocrine.
  Degenerative.
  Metabolic.
  Drugs.
- Pathophysiology.
- Clinical presentation.

- What would you do next?
- How would you manage this patient?
- What treatment options are available for this patient?
  - Conservative.
  - Medical.

- Radiological.
- Surgical.
- What is the overall prognosis?

Illustrative short cases

Case 1

You are asked to examine this patient.

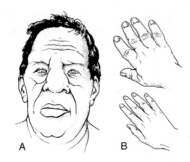

Q1: Please examine and describe the salient features of this patient.

Stand at the end of the patient's bed.

- **Inspection:** Look at the face.
  - Describe the coarse facial features – frontal bossing, large nose, prognathism.
  - Ask patient to open mouth, stick tongue out (large tongue) and to say 'arghh'. Coarse voice may be noted.
  - Examine hearing (e.g. conductive hearing loss).
- Ask to examine the hands.
  - Large and sweaty fingers.
  - Perform Tinel's and Phalen's tests.
  - Examine the ulnar nerve.
- At the end of the examination, you explain to the examiner: 'To complete the examination I would review the patient's blood pressure and pulse, assess the patient's visual fields and perform a urine dipstick test to check for glucose'.

Spot diagnosis: acromegaly.

Case 2
Q1: Please examine this patient's hands.

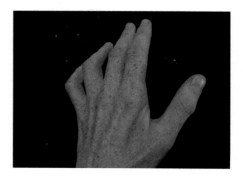

Inspection
- Place both hands on patient's lap or on a pillow.
- Compare both hands – dorsal and palmar aspects.
- Describe the wasting and weakness of the small muscles of the hand and partial clawing of the ring and little finger.
  - Comments – wasting of 1st dorsal interosseous muscle.
  - Finger clubbing (e.g. sign of Pancoast's tumour of the lung).
  - Petechial haemorrhages (e.g. vascular compromise – thoracic outlet syndrome).
- Ask patient to lift arms and then inspect medial epicondyle.
- Examine supracondylar region.

Power
- Dorsal interossei abducts the index, middle and ring fingers.
- Adductor digiti minimi abducts the little finger.
- Adductor pollicis adducts the thumb (e.g. Froment's sign).

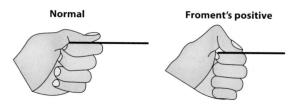

Normal	Froment's positive

- Flexor digitorum profundus flexes the wrist, metacarpophalangeal and interphalangeal joints.
- Flexor carpi ulnaris flexes and adducts the wrist joint.

Sensation
- Light touch and pinprick – assess medial 1½ fingers.

Differential diagnosis
- Ulnar nerve palsy.
- Brachial neuritis.
- Pancoast's syndrome.
- Thoracic outlet syndrome.

Spot diagnosis: ulnar nerve palsy.

Long cases

Common cases

- Pituitary tumours or sellar pathology.
  - Cushing.
  - Acromegaly.
  - Craniopharyngiomas.
- Cerebellopontine angle tumours.
  - Acoustic neuroma.
  - Neurofibromatosis 2.
  - Glomus jugulare tumours.
- Low-grade glioma.
- Radiation-induced meningioma.
- Cranio-cervical pathology.
- Syringomyelia.
- Chiari malformation.
- Meningioma.
- Spinal pathology.
- Von–Hippel Lindau syndrome.
- Brain stem cavernoma.
- Vascular.
  - Aneurysms.
  - Arteriovenous malformations (AVMs).
  - Carotid cavernous fistula (CCF).
- Benign intracranial hypertension (BIH).
- Normal pressure hydrocephalus (NPH).

History taking

Preparation

Ensure you take a targeted history in the allocated time allowed.

Introduce yourself to the patient.

Ensure adequate privacy.

You may ask the examiner to serve as your chaperone.

Targeted history taking

Obtain the patient's name, age, gender, handedness and occupation.

Establish the presenting complaint (PC).

Obtain the history of the presenting complaint (HPC).

- Chronological order of the symptoms: time course, onset, duration, frequency, progression, location, quality, quantity, severity, aggravating and relieving factors and associated symptoms.
- Risk factors for the presenting complaint.
- System-specific questions related to presenting complaint.
- Investigations and treatment provided to date.

Past medical/past surgical/past anaesthetic history (PMH/PSH/PAH)

- Use the mnemonic: THREADS MIJ.
  - **T**uberculosis.
  - **H**ypertension.
  - **R**heumatic fever/Rheumatoid arthritis.
  - **E**pilepsy.
  - **A**sthma.
  - **D**iabetes.
  - **S**troke.
  - **M**yocardial **I**nfarction.
  - **J**aundice.

Medication and known allergies

Note all medications that the patient is taking and any known allergies.

Family history (FH)

First-degree relatives with relevant familial diseases.

Social history (SH)

- Marital status.
- Occupation.
- Smoking habit (number of pack-years).
- Alcohol intake (units/week).
- Exposure to industrial toxins.
- Recreational drug use.
- Living accommodation.
- Level of support (family and carers).

Review of systems

During your targeted history taking, ask only the relevant questions based on the patient's history.

Cardiovascular system

Chest pain, dyspnoea, orthopnoea, palpitations, dizziness, ankle swelling.

Respiratory system

Dyspnoea, exercise tolerance, paroxysmal noctural dyspnoea, wheeze, chest pain, cough, haemoptysis, hoarseness, fever.

Gastrointestinal system

Change in appetite, diet regimen, weight loss (amount and duration), dysphasia, odynophagia, regurgitation of foods/liquids, indigestion, nausea, vomiting, haematemesis, abdominal pain, abdominal distention, change in bowel habit, rectal bleeding, flatulence, jaundice.

Urogenital system

Abdominal pain, frequency of micturition, dysuria, urgency, polyuria, colour of urine, haematuria, nocturia, impotence, sensation of incomplete voiding.

Central and peripheral nervous system

Fits, faints or funny turns, headache, loss of consciousness, tremor, muscle weakness, paralysis, sensory disturbances, paraesthesia, sphincter dysfunction, alteration in senses (smell, vision or hearing), change in behaviour or personality.

Musculoskeletal system

Muscle, bone or joint pain, deformity, swelling, stiffness, limb weakness, decreased range of movement, functional loss.

Metabolic system

Change in weight and appetite, alteration of build and appearance.

Summary

Use key words to describe the salient features.

Clinical examination

1. Introduction and consent

- Wash your hands.
- Introduce yourself to the patient and ask permission to examine him or her.
- Ensure adequate exposure of the patient.
- Check the patient's surroundings (e.g. walking or hearing aids, oxygen, drains, catheters, dressings).
- Inspect the patient as a whole (e.g. well – unwell/cachectic – obese/in pain – comfortable) including peripheral stigmata of underlying neurological disease, involuntary movements, abnormal facial expression.

2. Mental state evaluation

- **Appearance and behaviour.**
  Does the patient appear self-neglected, depressed or anxious; do they behave appropriately; have they experienced mood changes; are they appropriately concerned about their symptoms?
- **Mood.**
  Describe their current mood.
- **Systematic symptoms.**
  Is there a history of weight loss or gain, sleep disturbance, appetite changes, constipation, changes in libido or anxiety?
- **Delusion, hallucination and illusion.**
  Delusion: a firmly held belief, not altered by rational argument, and not based on conventional belief within a culture or society.
  Hallucination: a perception experienced without external stimuli that is indistinguishable from the perception of a real external stimulus.
  Illusion: a misinterpretation of an external stimulus.

3. Higher function evaluation

- **Attention and orientation.**
  Attention. Digital span: ask the patient to repeat a set of numbers (e.g. telephone number).

Orientation. Mini Mental State Examination (time, place, person).
- **Memory.**
  Immediate recall and attention.
  Name and address. Ask the patient to remember a specific name and address and ask the patient to immediately repeat it back to you.
  Short-term memory.
  After 5 minutes, ask the patient to recall the name and address.
  Long-term memory.
  Ask the patient to name the President of the United States or Prime Minister.
- **Calculation.**
  Serial sevens. Ask the patient to take 7 from 100, then 7 from 93 and so on.
- **Abstract thought (frontal lobe function).**
  Proverb. Ask the patient to explain a proverb: 'A stitch in times saves nine'.
- **Spatial perception (parietal and occipital lobe function).**
  Clock face. Ask the patient to draw a clock face and fill in the numbers. Then ask the patient to draw in the hands for the time 12:30 pm.
  Five-pointed star. Ask the patient to copy a five-pointed star.
- **Visual and body sensory perception (parietal and occipital function).**
  Recognize famous faces. Show the patient a picture of the President of the United States, Prime Minister or Queen.
  Body perception. Ask the patient to show the index finger and ring finger. Ask the patient to touch the right ear with the left index finger. Cross your hands and ask the patient which is your right hand.
  Sensory perception. Ask the patient to close the eyes. Write a number or letter on his or her hand and ask the patient to report the number or letter.
- **Apraxia.**
  Object recognition. Ask the patient to close their eyes. Place an object (e.g. coin, key, paper clip) in the patient's hand and ask him or her to identify the object.
  Three-hand test. Ask the patient to co~ your hand movements.

1. Make a fist and tap it on the table with your thumb facing upward.
2. Straighten out your fingers and tap on the table with your thumb facing upward.
3. Place your palm flat on the table.

4. Speech evaluation

To evaluate for dysphasia, first establish that there is no higher mental dysfunction or a confusional state. Exclude other speech disorders (e.g. dysarthria and dysphonia). To simplify, the different types of dysphasia are *expressive, receptive, conductive* and *dysnomial*. Expressive dysphasia is localized in the dominant posterior inferior frontal gyrus and frontal operculum (Broca's area). Receptive dysphasia is localized to the dominant posterior superior temporal gyrus and the inferior parietal lobule (Wernicke's area). Conductive dysphasia results from white matter tract disruption, located in the arcuate fasciculus. (Other tracts are being investigated.) It is worth noting that in a large number of postoperative cases, conductive dysphasia is common and likely to be assessed in this examination. Dysnomial dysphasia (inability to recall words or names) is not well localized. It may involve a breakdown in one or more pathways in different areas of the brain, including the parietal and temporal lobes.

The clinical evaluation of speech should be performed in quick and clear successive steps. Provide the examiner with a concluding statement at the end of each step.

Step 1: Ask the patient a question that requires a long and multi-sentenced answer.

Unless there is profound dysphasia, this step will assess higher mental function and orientation. It will be clear if the patient is suffering from an expressive dysphasia. Questions that are answered by short responses could potentially cause one to miss important speech deficits. For example, asking the patient to name various objects or colours is not sufficient.

Step 2: Determine whether the patient comprehends the complex task or discussion.

Do not rely on asking the patient to obey simple tasks, because you may miss a receptive dysphasia.

Step 3: Ask the patient to repeat a long sentence.

Repetition assesses for a conductive dysphasia, which is characterized by intact auditory comprehension, fluent speech production and poor speech repetition.

Step 4: Ask the patient to name certain objects.

Naming assesses for dysnomial dysphasia. The patient will have problems recalling words and names.

Step 5: Ask the patient to read a section of a newspaper or book.

Reading assesses for dyslexia. The patient will have an impaired ability to recognize and comprehend the written word. He or she may have difficulty in reading fluently, despite normal or above normal intelligence.

Step 6: Ask the patient to write a few sentences.

Writing assesses for dysgraphia. The patient will have difficulty writing (handwriting and possibly coherence).

Dysphasia

Receptive

Start with simple questions. Ask the patient to report his or her name, date and location.

Ask the patient to obey simple commands, such as close your eyes (visual command).

Expressive

Ask the patient to name objects, for instance, to describe what he or she eats for breakfast.

Repetition

Ask the patient to repeat 'no ifs, ands or buts' and 'the sun is shining'.

Reading

Ask the patient to read a sentence.

Writing

Ask the patient to write a simple sentence.

Dysarthria

Ask the patient to repeat: 'British constitution', 'West Register Street', and 'baby hippopotamus'.

Dysphonia

Ask the patient to cough and to say a sustained 'eeeeee'. Is there evidence of fatigue?

Listen to the patient's pitch, quality and tone of voice.

5. Lobe evaluation

Lobe evaluation is an essential component of the neurological examination.

   a. Frontal lobe.
   b. Parietal lobe.
   c. Temporal lobe.
   d. Occipital lobe.

a. Frontal lobe

Attention and orientation
Attention. Digital span: ask the patient to repeat a set of numbers (e.g. telephone number).
Orientation. Mini Mental State Examination (time, place, person).

Behaviour
Assess for apathy or disinhibition.

Abstract thought

Ask the patient to interpret 'A stich in time saves nine or 'A rolling stone gathers no moss'.

Motor

Ask patient to raise the arms. Assess for contralateral hemiplegia (e.g. pronator drift or motor weakness).

Speech

Broca's dysphasia (pars triangularis and pars opercularis of the inferior frontal gyrus): damage to this area results in expressive asphasia. Ask the patient to repeat: 'baby hippopotamus'.

Primitive reflexes

The primitive reflexes may be present.

- Palmar grasp reflex.
- Palmomental reflex.
- Rooting reflex.
- Glabellar reflex.

Frontal eye fields

Assess the patient's eye position in primary gaze position.
Assess the patient's extra-ocular eye movements, including saccadic eye movement.

Bladder function

Evidence of urinary urgency and incontinence.

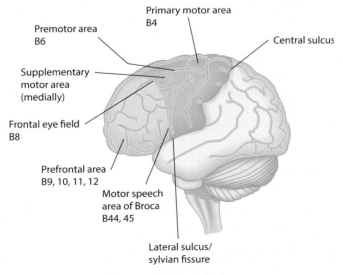

Figure 3.1 Frontal lobe

Sense of smell

Ask the patient if he or she has experienced a change or loss in sense of smell.

Gait

Assess for a 'magnetic' gait.

b. Parietal lobe

Establish the patient's dominant hand. This will enable the candidate to use the appropriate neurological examination for the affected area.

General function of parietal lobes (i.e. applicable to both hemispheres)
Cortical sensory function

- **Sensory perception.**
  - Ask the patient to close the eyes. Write a number or letter on the patient's hand and ask him or her to report the number or letter (e.g. graphaesthesia).
- **Tactile location/two-point discrimination.**
  - Ask the patient to close the eyes. Touch a certain point on the patient's skin surface. Then ask the patient to indicate the location of the previously touched point. The expected accuracy is a few millimetres on a fingertip and may be even 5–10 cm on the back.
  - Ask the patient to close the eyes. Use a caliper or a fashioned paper clip to touch one or two points. Ask the patient if he or she feels 'one' or 'two' points.
- **Stereognosis.**
  - Ask the patient to close the eyes. Ask the patient to identify objects (e.g. coin and key) in each hand (**astereognosia** – inability to perform this action).
- **Tactile extinction (sensory inattention).**
  - Test individual body parts on opposite sides of the body and simultaneously. Ask the patient to close the eyes, then touch the patient on both sides of the body, simultaneously initially and then alternately. Ask the patient to tell you when you are touching him or her (e.g. right hand; both hands; and left face and right hand). To make the test more sensitive, test different body parts at the same time (e.g. face and hand).
  - Patient ignores or denies any neurological deficit on the affected contralateral side of the body (hemi-asomatognosia, sensory neglect).

Visual fields

Assess for a homonymous hemianopia.

Specific function of parietal lobe (depending on hemispheric dominance)
1. In the dominant hemisphere

Gerstmann's syndrome – dominant parietal lobe.	
Left-right dissociation	cross your hands and ask the patient which hand is right and left.
Acalculia	patient is unable to perform calculations – serial 7s.
Agraphia	patient is unable to write.
Finger agnosia	patient is unable to distinguish fingers [left index from left thumb].

Left-right disorientation

Ask patient to touch their right ear with the left thumb.

Calculation
Serial sevens.

Ask the patient to take 7 from 100, then 7 from 93, and so on.

Finger agnosia

Ask the patient to show the index finger and ring finger. Ask patient to name fingers (finger agnosia).

Dyspraxia (ideo, ideomotor and motor)
Three-hand test.

Ask the patient to copy your hand movements.

1. Make a fist and tap it on the table with your thumb facing upward.
2. Straighten out your fingers and tap on the table with your thumb facing upward.
3. Then place your palm flat on the table.

Activities of daily living (ideomotor apraxia).

Ask patient to comb their hair, drink a cup of tea, or strike a match and blow it out.

2. In the non-dominant hemisphere

Spatial perception (parietal and occipital lobe function)

- **Clock face.** Ask the patient to draw a clock face and fill in the numbers. Then ask the patient to draw in the hands for the time: e.g. 12:30 pm.
- **Five-pointed star.** Ask the patient to copy a five-pointed star.

Geographical dyspraxia

- Patient is unable to locate defined places or known locations.

Motor

Ask the patient if he or she has a history of difficulties swallowing (oral stage).

Combination of functions with other lobes
Attention and orientation (frontal, parietal, temporal and occipital lobes)

Attention. Digital span: ask the patient to repeat a set of numbers (e.g. telephone number).
Orientation. Mini Mental State Examination (time, place, person).

Visual and body sensory perception (parietal and occipital function)
Recognize famous faces.

- Show the patient a picture of the President of the United States, Prime Minster or Queen.
- Ask the patient to touch their right ear with the left index finger.
- Cross your hands and ask the patient which is your right hand.

c. Temporal lobe

Attention and orientation

Attention. Digital span: ask the patient to repeat a set of numbers (e.g. telephone number).
Orientation. Mini Mental State Examination (time, place, person).

Memory

Assess for impaired immediate recall and attention. Name and address: Ask the patient to remember a name and address and ask the patient to immediately repeat it back to you.

Assess for impaired short-term memory. After 5 minutes ask the patient to recall the name and address.

Assess for impaired long-term memory. Name of President of the United States or Prime Minister.

Speech

Wernicke's dysphasia (posterior part of the superior temporal gyrus): damage to this area results in a receptive aphasia. The patient is unable to understanding what has been said, e.g. unable to execute commands. Ask the patient to follow a command: 'When I clap my hands, and not before, touch your left ear with your right hand'. Note that the command must be delivered with no non-verbal communication. Also, beware of underlying hemiplegia.

Hearing

Assess the auditory cortex, which includes the superior temporal gyrus, within the lateral fissure and composes parts of Heschl's gyrus and the superior temporal gyrus, including the planum polare and temporale (only in suspected cases of bitemporal temporal lobe involvement). Be aware that hearing is bilaterally represented in the cortex.

Visual fields

Visual field (the optic radiation or geniculo-calcarine tract) defects result from damage to Meyer's loop resulting a superior quadrantanopia ('pie in the sky') and loss of colour vision.

d. Occipital lobe

Visual fields

- If one occipital lobe is damaged, this can result in a homonymous hemianopsia.
- Occipital lesions may also cause visual hallucinations.
- Lesions in the parietal-temporal-occipital association area are associated with colour agnosia, movement agnosia, and agraphia.
- Damage to the primary visual cortex, which is located on the surface of the posterior occipital lobe, can lead to blindness.

Combined functions with other lobes
Attention and orientation

Attention. Digital span: ask the patient to repeat a set of numbers (e.g. telephone number).

Orientation. Mini Mental State Examination (time, place, person).

Spatial perception (a combination of parietal and occipital lobe function)

- **Clock face.** Ask the patient to draw a clock face and fill in the numbers. Then ask the patient to draw in the hands for the time: e.g. 12:30 pm.
- **Five-pointed star.** Ask the patient to copy a five-pointed star.

Visual and body sensory perception (parietal and occipital function)

- **Recognize famous faces.** Show the patient a picture of the President of the United States, Prime Minister or Queen.
- **Body perception.**
  - Ask the patient to show the index finger and ring finger.
  - Ask the patient to touch the right ear with the left index finger.
  - Cross your hands and ask the patient which is your right hand.
- **Sensory perception.** Ask the patient to close the eyes. Write a number or letter on the patient's hand and ask him or her to report the number or letter.

Illustrative cases
Case 1
A 64-year-old woman presents with a 5-year history of personality change and is now admitted with a generalized seizure.

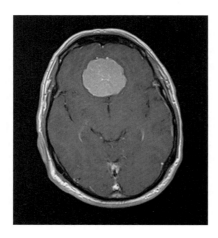

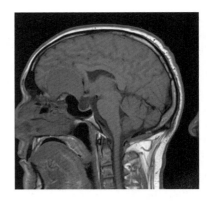

Q1: What is the likely diagnosis?

This MRI scan demonstrates a large well-defined mass with mild surrounding oedema in the inter-hemispheric fissure of the frontal lobe. These features are suggestive of an olfactory groove meningioma.

Q2: With this in mind, demonstrate the relevant positive neurological signs.

Because the MRI scan demonstrates a medial frontal lobe lesion, it is appropriate to proceed with a general examination followed by a focussed evaluation of the frontal lobe and cranial nerves (including the olfactory and optic nerves).

Inspection
- Appearance and behaviour.
- Comments about the position of the patient's eyes.
- Assess for saccadic eye movement (frontal eye fields).

Ask the patient a few brief questions
- MMS (time, place, person).
- Interpret 'A rolling stone gathers no moss' (abstract thinking).
- Ask about sense of smell.
- Ask about bladder function.

Ask patient to raise their arms
- Comments about pronator drift or motor weakness.
- Elicit grasp reflex.
- Pout reflex.
- Palmomental reflex.

Assess the patient's gait and mobility

Case 2

A 58-year-old experienced mathematics teacher has recent problems with reduced concentration and intermittent headaches. There is disruption in his classroom during lessons. An MRI scan is arranged.

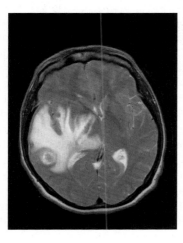

Q1: Perform a focussed relevant examination for this patient.

Introduce yourself and ask permission to examine the patient.

Inspection

Comment about the patient's facial appearance (e.g. facial palsy) and general demeanour.

Ask patient a few brief questions

- Hand dominance.

Assess the patient's speech

Ask the patient to follow the following instructions

- Touch the nose with the left index finger (left-right disorientation).
- Name the fingers (finger agnosia).
- Ask the patient to perform mathematics – serial sevens (dyscalculia).
- Read and write.

Ask patient to lift their arms

- Comments about pronator drift or motor weakness.
- Pretend to write number on the palm of the hand (agraphastesia).
- Place coin in palm (astereognosia).
- Test for sensation/neglect (sensory inattention).
- Two-point discrimination.

Ask patient to perform the following tasks

- Comb hair, drink a cup of tea, strike a match and blow it out (dominant hemisphere) (ideo-motor apraxia).
- Ask the patient to draw clock face or 5-pointed star (constructional apraxia).

Ask whether patient has any difficulty finding his/her way around familiar places (geographical apraxia)

Assess the patient's visual fields

Q2: What is the reason for the disruption in his classroom?

This is attributed to a combination of dysphasia and difficulty with dyscalculia.

6. Central nervous system evaluation

Detailed cranial nerve (I–XII) examination

Inspection: involuntary movements (tremor, choreiform movement), dysphasia (expressive and receptive) and abnormal facial movements (facial weakness, ptosis).

When asked to examine the eyes begin by asking the patient if he or she can see with both eyes. If the patient is blind in one eye, then it would be inappropriate to cover the blind eye when examining the visual fields. The two main components of this examination are the assessment of the optic nerve (**cranial nerve II**) and of the eye movements (**cranial nerves III, IV, VI**).

Start by examining the direct and consensual light reflex and accommodation. Perform swinging light test to assess for a relative afferent pupillary defect (RAPD) only if it is indicated. This defect is more likely to be present in patients with poor vision in one eye (another good reason to have asked the patient about vision prior to the start of this examination). The one pitfall includes bringing the light torch into the patient's field of view while shining the light because the pupillary reaction could result in accommodation rather than assessing the light reflex.

When assessing visual acuity ensure that the patient is at the correct distance from the Snellen chart. In addition, you should not hold the reading chart, such as the Jaeger chart, but rather let the patient hold it at his or her reading distance.

To examine visual fields by confrontation, ensure that the hat pin is equidistant between yourself and the patient. Assess for an enlarged blind spot. There is debate on whether the hat pin should be red or white. A loss of red colour vision occurs early in lesions of the optic nerve and optic chiasm. A red hat pin is a sensitive way to detect defects as a result of pathological processes in this region of the pituitary and suprasellar fossa. When you are examining for a retrochiasmatic lesion (e.g. homonymous hemianopia), the red colour becomes irrelevant.

During this part of the examination, there can be major challenges. The visual fields of both eyes overlap; therefore each eye is tested independently. The patient should cover the right eye with the right hand (vice versa when testing the opposite eye). A better technique is to cover the patient's right eye while you close your right eye. By performing this manoeuvre, you will be at arm's length and equidistant to the patient. Use a red hat pin as the moving target. Start outside the usual 180° visual field, then move slowly to a more central position until the patient confirms visualization of the target. All four quadrants (upper and lower, temporal and nasal) should be tested. When you switch from temporal to nasal fields, swap your covering hands to avoid your arms crossing in front of the patient. If the object is nearer to the patient than to you, you will detect a visual field defect that does not exist. Remember, it is unlikely to see an enlarged blind spot without papilloedema or a degree of optic atrophy.

While examining the eyes, if you detect a visual field defect, it is important to examine cranial nerves III, IV and VI. In cases of pituitary macroadenoma invading the cavernous sinus, these cranial nerves may all be involved. If the question was specifically to examine the eye movements, then take your time to complete this task. Similarly during fundoscopy, if the examiner does not report that the fundi are normal and prompts you to move forward, take your time to inspect both fundi because an abnormality may be present.

When examining eye movements, include the assessment of pursuit and saccadic movements and presence of nystagmus. Ask the patient to report diplopia (double vision), because failure to talk to the patient during examination may lead to incomplete illustration of the underlying deficit. If there is evidence of uncoordinated movements without diplopia, ask the patient if he or she has been diagnosed with a squint. In patients with diplopia, cover alternate eyes to establish which suppresses the false image. This is important to differentiate between subtle abduction palsy in one eye and limited adduction in the other eye. When you report your findings to the examiner, explain the movement's deficit rather than the cranial nerve. For example, limited abduction is called abduction palsy. This could originate from a VI cranial nerve palsy or mechanical reason in the orbit. A complete IV cranial nerve palsy will result in a characteristic 'down and out' position in the affected eye. Patients report difficulty looking down when coming down a staircase.

Internuclear ophthalmoplegia (INO), or the 'one and a half syndrome', which is more common in patients with multiple sclerosis, is a disorder of conjugate lateral gaze in which the affected eye shows impaired adduction. When an attempt is made to gaze contralaterally (relative to the affected eye), the affected eye adducts minimally, if at all. The contralateral eye abducts with nystagmus. Additionally, the divergence of the eyes leads to horizontal diplopia. Convergence is generally preserved.

Once you have detected a defect, perform further cranial nerve examination. If you confirm an ophthalmoplegia then examine the trigeminal nerve to exclude a possible cavernous sinus lesion.

If upward gaze is limited, examine for Parinaud's syndrome (dorsal midbrain syndrome). There will be abnormalities of eye movement and pupil function. The syndrome is characterized by upward gaze limitation, pseudo-Argyll Robertson pupils (accommodative paresis ensues, and the pupils become mid-dilated and show light-near dissociation), convergence-retraction nystagmus (nystagmus rectactorius), eyelid retraction (Collier's sign) and a conjugate downgaze in the neutral position ('setting-sun' sign).

If the examiner instructs you to examine the lower cranial nerves, start with cranial nerves V–VIII, bearing in mind the fact that if there are no detected abnormalities, then move directly to cranial nerves IX–XII.

Examination of **cranial nerve V** is straightforward. The time taken for this examination is variable. The most sensitive test for cranial nerve V dysfunction is the loss of corneal reflex. (This is usually the only deficit even with a large trigeminal schwannoma.) In cases where you do not detect a blink reflex, ask the patient whether he or she can feel the stimulus. If the patient wears contact lenses, the blink reflex would be absent bilaterally. When testing the sensory branches of the cranial nerve V, it is important to apply the stimulus to each division (ophthalmic, maxillary and mandibular branches). For testing sensation in the maxillary division, apply the stimulus near the nasolabial fold or on the midline of the cheek. For testing sensation over the mandibular division, apply the stimulus on the anterior chin nearest to the midline. Avoid the skin over the angle of the mandible because this can also be supplied by the upper cervical cutaneous nerves. When testing for light touch and pinprick in the

three divisions, a discrete lesion in the brainstem may only affect one modality. In cases of central brainstem lesions such as syringobulbia, patients may present with an appearance of an 'onion peel', 'onion skin' or a 'balaclava helmet'. Examination of the motor component of cranial nerve V should be quick. Palpate for the contraction of the masseter while the patient clenches the teeth, then assess lateral lower jaw movements against resistance.

Examination of **cranial nerve VII** involves an assessment of motor and sensory testing. Ask the patient to perform the following manoeuvres: raise the eyebrows (frontalis muscle supplied by temporal branch of facial nerve), frown, and close the eyes (orbicularis oculi) with or without a Bell's phenomenon. If the eye closure is incomplete, examine the corneal reflex (cranial nerve V). If both cranial V and VII are absent, there is an increased risk of corneal ulceration, and you should consider a partial tarsorraphy. Assess lower facial movements by asking the patient to smile, blow out the cheeks and whistle. Once you detect a facial nerve palsy, assess for surgical or post-operative causes by examining for craniotomy scars.

Examination of **cranial nerve VIII** includes an assessment of hearing and balance. Begin by asking the patient if he or she has diminished hearing in one ear. Without this information, the interpretation of tuning fork tests will be complex. Inspect the ear canal and tympanic membrane to ensure that there is no obstruction or perforation. Use the appropriate tuning fork frequency (512 Hz) for the hearing tests. The tuning fork for vibration is 128 Hz.

Examination of **cranial nerves IX and X** is important. Glossopharyngeal nerve lesions can produce the following: difficulty swallowing; impairment of taste over the posterior one-third of the tongue and palate; impaired sensation over the posterior one-third of the tongue, palate, and pharynx; an absent gag reflex; and dysfunction of the parotid gland. Vagus nerve lesions produce palatal and pharyngeal paralysis; laryngeal paralysis; abnormalities of oesophageal motility, gastric acid secretion, gallbladder emptying, and heart rate; and other autonomic dysfunction. Begin by testing the patient's gag reflex. In cases of an absent gag reflex and/or deviation of the uvula (away from the side of the lesion) while asking the patient to say 'ah', indicate dysfunction of the IX–XI cranial nerves. If the gag reflex is absent, assess if the patient has preserved sensation on both sides of the oropharynx. Occasionally patients who have worn dentures for a long time may lose the gag reflex although the pharyngeal sensation remains intact. Ask the patient to cough and note if a hoarse voice is present. If the lateral sign is present, consider further assessment by formal laryngoscopy.

Examination of **cranial nerve XI** assesses the actions of trapezius and sternocleidomastoid muscles. Observe the volume and contour of the sternocleidomastoid muscles as the patient looks straight ahead. Test the right sternocleidomastoid muscle by facing the patient and placing your right palm laterally on the patient's left cheek. Ask the patient to turn the head to the left, resisting the pressure you are exerting in the opposite direction. At the same time, observe and palpate the right sternocleidomastoid with your left hand. Then reverse the procedure to test the left sternocleidomastoid. Now test the trapezius muscle. Ask the patient to face away from you. Observe the shoulder contour for hollowing, displacement or winging of the scapula and drooping of the shoulder. Place your hands on the patient's shoulders and press down as the patient shrugs the shoulders and then retracts.

The examination of **cranial nerve XII** starts by inspecting the tongue with the opened mouth while the tongue remains within the oral cavity. Fasiculations are reliably detected before tongue protrusion. If there is cranial nerve palsy on protruding the tongue, it becomes deviated toward the side of lesion as a result of weakness of the action of the genioglossus muscle. Movements from side to side against the resistance of the cheeks would detect more subtle weakness. If there is significant weakness, assess for hemiatrophy, which reflects the longstanding nature of this deficit.

Summary of cranial nerve (I-XII) examination

I Olfactory

Assess the patient's sense of smell by testing each nostril in turn. Use essence bottles of coffee, vanilla and peppermint.

II Optic

General: observe for pupil asymmetry, ptosis and swelling.

Visual acuity: if the patient wears glasses, keep them on. Test each eye separately using a Snellen chart.

Visual fields: stand 2 feet in front of the patient and ensure you are at eye level. Move your hands to the side halfway between yourself and the patient, wiggle fingers and ask the patient when he or she sees movement. Assess nasal and temporal fields.

Fundoscopy: assess the fundus, macula and optic disc.

III, IV VI Oculomotor, Trochlear, Abducens

Inspect the pupils: shape and presence of ptosis.

Pupil reaction: to light (direct, consensual and swinging light test) and accommodation.

Extra-ocular eye movements: assess saccadic and pursuit eye movements.

V Trigeminal

Facial sensation: forehead, cheek and jaw.

Motor: assess the following muscles: temporalis, masseter, pterygoids.

Ask the patient to open their mouth and clench their teeth.

Assess bite strength.

Assess corneal reflex.

Assess jaw jerk.

VII Facial

Inspect for facial droop or asymmetry.

Facial expression: ask the patient to look up and wrinkle their forehead. Inspect for wrinkle loss. Ask the patient to shut their eyes tightly. Ask the patient to smile and look for asymmetry in the patient's nasolabial folds. In addition, ask the patient to frown, show their teeth and puff out their cheeks. Assess for taste.

VIII Vestibulocochlear

Auditory acuity of each ear: Place your hands by each of the patient's ears. Rub your fingers to create noise on one side, and keep the other hand still. Then switch hands. Ask the patient from which ear the noise is heard. If hearing loss is identified, inspect the external auditory canals and the tympanic membranes.

Rinne's test (air vs. bone conduction).
Apply tuning fork (512 Hz) on the mastoid behind the ear. Ask the patient when he or she can no longer hear the sound. Then move the tuning fork next to the patient's ear canal so he or she can hear the sound. A normal response is that air conduction (ear) is better heard than bone conduction (mastoid).
Weber's test (lateralization).
Apply tuning fork (256 Hz) to the top of patient's head on the middle of the forehead. Ask the patient 'where do you hear the sound coming from?' A normal response is in the midline.
Test oculocephalic reflex (doll's eye manoeuvre).
Test oculovestibular reflex (ear canal caloric stimulation).

IX, X Glossopharygeal, Vagus

Assess the patient's voice for hoarseness.
Ask the patient to swallow and cough.
Examine the palate for uvular displacement.
Assess the soft palate movement by asking the patient to say 'ah'.
Perform the gag reflex.

XI Accessory

Examine for atrophy and asymmetry of the trapezius muscle.
Ask the patient to shrug their shoulders.
Turn the patient's head against resistance, inspect and palpate the sternocleidomastoid muscle.

XII Hypoglossal

Listen to articulation.
Inspect the patient's tongue for wasting or fasciculations.
Ask the patient to protrude the tongue: the tongue will deviate to the affected side.

The timing and speed of your cranial nerve examination is of utmost importance. A slow examination results in a missed opportunity to examine other clinical cases and gives the impression that you are inexperienced and lack confidence. A hasty examination may result in the omission of key important signs.

7. Cerebellar evaluation

Cerebellar dysfunction is assessed by using the mnemonic DANISH:

- **D**ysdiadochokinesia. Ask the patient to rapidly pronate and supinate their hand on the opposite side. Repeat with the other hand. The patient will have an inability to perform rapid alternating movements.
- **A**taxia. Assess for a broad-based unsteady gait with lumbering movements. The patient may demonstrate variable distance between steps and difficulty with turning.
- **N**ystagmus. Assess for oscillating eye movements.
- **I**ntention tremor. Ask the patient to point from their nose to your finger. Ensure your finger is at arm's length, and then move your finger to different places. As the patient's finger approaches your finger, a tremor may be noticed or there may be evidence of past pointing.
- **S**taccato speech. Ask the patient to repeat 'British constitution' or 'pink hippopotamus'.
- **H**ypotonia. Assess for reduced tone in the patient's upper and lower limbs.

8. Gait evaluation

- **Walking:** initiation, gait symmetry, size of paces, posture, arms swing, turning, speed, fluency of stepping, stride length, distance between feet (base). Also inspect the patient's knees, pelvis and shoulders.
- **Inspect the patient's shoes.**
- **Ask the patient to heel-to-toe walk (as if on a tightrope), walk on their toes and heels.**
- **Romberg test** (to assess the dorsal columns of the spinal cord): ask the patient to stand with the feet together and ask the patient to close their eyes.

9. Peripheral nervous system evaluation (upper and lower limbs)

Tone, power, coordination, sensation (light touch, pinprick, temperature, proprioception, vibration, two-point discrimination) and reflexes.

Upper limb examination

Introduce and ask permission to examine patient.
Expose the upper limbs.
Comment on the patient's surroundings (hand splints, medication).
Detailed inspection.
  Inspect the patient as a whole (e.g. well/unwell/cachectic/pain-free/in pain).
  Inspect for the following: Asymmetry, deformities, scars, tremor, muscle wasting, fasciculations, involuntary movements, peripheral stigmata of underlying neurological disease and supraclavicular fullness.
Muscle tone.
  Ask the patient whether there is any pain.
  Roll arm in clockwise and counterclockwise direction. Assess for rigidity. Test for clonus.
Power.
  Ask the patient to raise the arms. Comment on evidence of a pronator drift or limb weakness.

MRC Grade	
5/5	Normal: movement against gravity – full power
4/5	Movement against specific gravity and resistance, but weaker than normal
3/5	Movement against gravity
2/5	Movement with gravity eliminated
1/5	Visible contraction, but no movement
0/5	No contraction

Myotomes		
Root	Reflex	Movement
C5	Biceps	Elbow flexion, shoulder abduction
C6	Supinator	Elbow flexion (semi pronated)
C7	Triceps	Elbow extension, finger extension
C8	Finger	Finger flexion
T1	No reflex	Small muscles of the hand

The radial nerve and its branches supply all extension in the arm.

The median nerve supplies the LOAF muscles (lateral two lumbricals, opponens pollics, abductor pollicis brevis, flexor pollicis brevis).

The ulnar nerve supplies all intrinsic hand muscles except the LOAF muscles.

Coordination.
  • Finger – nose test.
Sensation.
  • Fine touch.

Root	Location
C5	Shoulder
C6	Lateral arm/thumb
C7	Back of hand
C8	Medial hand
T1	Medial arm

  • Pinprick.
  • Temperature.
  • Two-point discrimination.
  • Joint position sense (shoulder, elbow, finger).
  • Vibration sense (sternum, wrist, elbow, shoulder).

Reflexes.
  • Biceps (C5, C6).
  • Supinator (C5, C6).
  • Triceps (C6, C7).
  • Finger flexors – Hoffmann's sign.
  • Pectoral reflex.
  • Deltoid reflex.

Reflexes are graded using a 0 to 4+ scale.

Grade	Description
0	Absent
1+	Hypoactive
2+	Normal
3+	Hyperactive without clonus
4+	Hyperactive with clonus

Complete the upper limb examination.
- Examine the patient's spine.
- Examine the cranial nerves and neurology of the lower limbs.

Arrange for appropriate investigations.
- Bedside tests (e.g. observation charts, dipstick urine, ECG).
- Bloods (e.g. group and save, FBC, U&E, CRP).
- Radiological imaging (e.g. radiographs, CT scan and MRI scan).
- Special tests (e.g. EEG, nerve conduction studies, PET scan).

Treatment options.
- Conservative.
- Medical.
- Radiological.
- Surgical.

Lower limb examination

Introduce yourself and ask permission to examine patient.
Expose the lower limbs.
Comment on the patient's surroundings (leg splints, medication).
Detailed inspection.
  Inspect the patient as a whole (e.g. well/unwell/cachectic/pain-free/in pain).
  Inspect for the following:
    Asymmetry, deformities, scars, tremor, muscle wasting, fasciculations, involuntary movements, peripheral stigmata of underlying neurological disease.
    Assess the back for deformity or scars.

Gait.
  Ask the patient to walk to a fixed point, walk heel – toe and walk on heels and toes.
  Inspect patient's shoes.
  Comment on the patient's posture.
  Perform Romberg's test.
Muscle tone.
  Ask the patient whether there is any pain.
  Roll the legs, lift and release the knees. Assess for rigidity.
  Test for clonus.
Power.
  Ask the patient to lift the legs. Comment on evidence of limb weakness.

MRC Grade	
5/5	Normal: movement against gravity – full power
4/5	Movement against specific gravity and resistance, but weaker than normal
3/5	Movement against gravity
2/5	Movement with gravity eliminated
1/5	Visible contraction, but no movement
0/5	No contraction

Myotomes		
Root	Reflex	Movement
L1,L2	No reflex	Hip flexion
L3,L4	Knee reflex	Knee extension
L5	No reflex	Dorsiflexion of foot, inversion and eversion of ankle, extension of great toe
S1	Ankle reflex	Hip extension, knee extension, plantarflexion

Coordination.
- Heel-shin test.

Sensation.
- Fine touch.

Root	Location
L1	Inguinal area
L2,3	Anterior thigh
L4,L5	Shin
S1	Lateral foot and sole

- Pinprick.
- Temperature.
- Two-point discrimination.
- Joint position sense (hip, knee, toes).
- Vibration sense (ankle, tibial tuberosity, iliac crest).

Reflexes.
- Knee (L3, L4).
- Ankle (L5, S1).
- Plantar reflex: Babinski (extensor).

Reflexes are graded using a 0 to 4+ scale:

Grade	Description
0	Absent
1+	Hypoactive
2+	Normal
3+	Hyperactive without clonus
4+	Hyperactive with clonus

Complete the lower limb examination.
- Examine the patient's spine.
- Examine the cranial nerves and neurology of the upper limbs.

Arrange for appropriate investigations.
- Bedside tests (e.g. observation charts, dipstick urine, ECG).
- Bloods (e.g. group and save, FBC, U&E, CRP).
- Radiological imaging (e.g. radiographs, CT scan and MRI scan).
- Special tests (e.g. EEG, nerve conduction studies, PET scan).

Treatment options.
- Conservative.
- Medical.
- Radiological.
- Surgical.

10. Neurocutaneous syndrome evaluation

The diagnosis is made on clinical history and examination and confirmed by diagnostic testing.

The most common types of neurocutaneous syndromes are the following:

1. Tuberous sclerosis (TS).
2. Neurofibromatosis types 1 and 2.
3. Von Hippel–Lindau disease.
4. Sturge–Weber disease.
5. Osler–Weber Rendu syndrome.

1. Tuberous sclerosis: clinical presentation

A 23-year-old man presents with a 3-year history of headaches, which have progressed over the past 1–2 months. In addition, he presents with symptoms of nausea and vomiting. His past medical history includes seizures, which resolved when he was 10 years of age.

Tuberous sclerosis is a rare multi-system genetic disease (autosomal dominant) characterized by hamartomas of many organs including skin, brain, eyes, kidneys, heart and lungs. The combination of symptoms includes seizures, intellectual disability, developmental delay, behavioural problems, skin abnormalities and diseases of the lung and kidney. It is caused by mutation of either of two genes, *TSC1* (chromosome 9) and *TSC2* (chromosome 16), which code for the proteins hamartin and tuberin respectively. These proteins act as tumour growth suppressors.

The classic clinical triad consists of seizures, mental retardation and sebaceous adenomas.

Patients present with the following:
- Facial angiofibromas.
- Periungual and subungal fibromas.
- Fibrous plaques of the forehead and scalp.

Associated conditions include the following:
- Tubers.
- Subependymal giant cell astrocytoma (SEGA).

- Multiple calcified subependymal nodules.
- Multiple retinal astrocytomas.
- Retinal hamartomas or achromic patch.
- Shagreen patch.
- Pulmonary lymphangiomyomatosis.
- Renal angiomyolipoma.
- Renal cysts.
- Cardiac rhabdomyomas.

2. Neurofibromatosis (1 and 2): clinical presentation

A 29-year-old left-handed woman presents with unilateral hearing loss and tinnitus. Moreover, she presents with reduced visual acuity and diplopia.

Neurofibromatosis (NFT) refers to a number of inherited conditions that are clinically and genetically distinct and carry a high risk of tumour formation, particularly in the brain. Neurofibromatosis is an autosomal dominant condition. The severity in affected individuals can vary; this may be due to variable expression. Approximately half of cases are due to *de novo* mutations and no other affected family members are seen.

Neurofibromatosis 1 (>90% of cases of neurofibromatosis), chromosome 17q11.2 which codes for neurofibromin.

1. Six or more café-au-lait spots (≥ 0.5 cm in prepubertal subjects or ≥ 1.5 cm in postpuberta subjects). ·
2. ≥ 2 neurofibromas or one plexiform neurofibroma.
3. Freckling in the axilla or groin.
4. Optic glioma.
5. Two or more Lisch nodules.
6. A distinctive bony lesion (dysplasia of the sphenoid bone or dysplasia or thinning of long bone cortex).
7. A first-degree relative with NFT-1.

Associated conditions.
- Schwann cell tumours on any nerve.
- Spinal +/– peripheral nerve neurofibromas.
- Multiple skin neurofibromas.
- Aqueductal stenosis.
- Macrocephaly.

- Intracranial tumours: astroctyomas, mengingiomas.
- Optic glioma.
- Kyphoscoliosis.
- Syringomyelia.
- Malignant tumours: neuroblastoma, ganglioma, sarcoma, leukaemia, Wilm's tumour.
- Phaechromocytoma.
- Mental retardation.
- Learning difficulties.

Neurofibromatosis 2, chromosome 22q12.2 which results in the inactivation of schwannomin.

1. Bilateral vestibular schwannomas.
2. OR first degree relative with NFT-2 and either:
   A. unilateral eight nerve mass.
   B. OR two of the following.
      1. Neurofibroma.
      2. Meningioma.
      3. Glioma: includes astrocytoma, ependymoma.
      4. Schwannomas: including spinal root schwannoma.
      5. Juvenile posterior subcapsular lenticular opacities or cataract.

Associated conditions include the following:
- Seizures.
- Skin nodules, dermal neurofibromas, café au lait spots (less common than NFT-1).
- Multiple intradural spinal tumours (less common in NFT-1) including intramedullary (ependymomas) and extramedullary (schwannomas, meningioma) tumours.
- Antigenic nerve growth factor is increased.

3. Von Hippel Lindau disease: clinical presentation

A 36-year-old man presents with nausea, vomiting and headaches for 1 week. His MRI scan demonstrates a dilated fourth ventricle with a cystic lesion in the left cerebellar hemisphere.

Von Hippel–Lindau (VHL) disease is a rare autosomal dominant genetic condition that predisposes individuals to benign and malignant tumours. VHL results from a mutation in the von Hippel–Lindau tumour suppressor gene on chromosome 3p25.3.

1. One or more haemangioblastomas (HGBs) within the central nervous system (CNS) (typically a cerebellar HGB and a retinal HGB and angioma).
2. Inconstant presence of visceral lesions (usually renal +/– pancreatic tumours or cysts).
3. Frequent familial incidence.

Associated conditions

- Haemangioblastomas of the cerebellum and spinal cord.
- Retinal angiomas.
- Retinal haemangioblastomas.
- Renal cell carcinomas.
- Pheochromocytomas.
- Polycythemia.
- Cysts (hepatic, renal, pancreas and epididymal).
- Endolymphatic sac tumour.
- Epididymal papillary cystadenomas.

4. Sturge–Weber syndrome: clinical presentation

A 34-year-old man presents with a grand mal seizure while at work. He suffers from long-standing epilepsy and headaches.

Sturge–Weber syndrome is a rare congenital neurological and skin disorder. It is often associated with port-wine stains of the face, glaucoma, seizures, mental retardation, and ipsilateral leptomeningeal angioma. It is characterized by abnormal blood vessels on the brain surface. Normally, only one side of the brain is affected. Sturge–Weber is an embryonal developmental anomaly resulting from errors in mesodermal and ectodermal development. Most cases are sporadic. It is caused by a somatic activating mutation occurring in the GNAQ gene.

A. Localized cerebral cortical atrophy and calcifications (especially layers 2 and 3, with a predilection for the occipital lobes):
1. Calcifications appear as curvilinear double parallel lines ('tram tracking') on plain X-rays.
2. Cortical atrophy usually causes contralateral haemiparesis, haemiatrophy, and homonymous haemianopia (with occipital lobe involvement).

B. Ipsilateral port-wine facial nevus (nevus flammeus) usually in distribution of the ophthalmic division of trigeminal nerve).

Associated conditions

- Ipsilateral exophthalmos +/– glaucoma, coloboma of the iris.
- Oculomeningeal capillary haemangioma.
- Convulsive seizures (contralateral to the facial nevus and cortical atrophy).
- Retinal angioma.
- Haemiparesis.
- Mental retardation.
- Learning disability.
- Developmental delay.
- Haemianopsia.
- Vascular headaches.
- Moyamoya disease.
- Arteriovenous malformations of the lung and liver.

5. Osler–Weber Rendu syndrome: clinical presentation

A 53-year-old woman presents with recurrent epistaxis, which requires repeated hospital admissions.

Osler–Weber Rendu syndrome (hereditary haemorrhagic telangiectasia [HHT]) is a rare autosomal dominant genetic disorder that is linked to tumour growth factor B (TGF-B), HHTL (endoglin, chromosome 9) and HHT2 (ALK1, chromosome 12). Haploinsufficiency leads to a deficiency in angiogenesis. This leads to abnormal blood vessel formation in the skin, in the mucous membranes, and often in organs such as the lungs, liver and brain.

Associated conditions

- Recurrent epistaxis.
- Cerebrovascular malformations including telangiectasia, AVMs, venous angiomas and aneurysms.
- Pulmonary arteriovenous fistulas with risk of paradoxical cerebral embolism, which predisposes to embolic stroke and cerebral abscess.

4

The viva: operative surgery and surgical anatomy

Because this book is a guide to the neurosurgical examination, this chapter is not intended to serve as an operative textbook. This guide identifies the examination 'favourites'. During the operative and surgical anatomy viva, convey your personal experience rather than reciting a surgical textbook. Throughout this chapter, short tables are added to alert the reader about important key points and potential challenging areas of discussion. The selected procedures are not an exhaustive list, but rather demonstrate common principles that can be applied in presenting a variety of operations in the examination setting. For some important procedures, the emphasis is on the surgical principles and specific points that are likely to be asked. This is to remind the reader that it is important to understand the basic principles of auxiliary aids in surgery (e.g. technical equipment and instruments, intraoperative dyes, neurophysiological intraoperative monitoring, angiographic planning in vascular cases, special anaesthetic techniques) because they are likely to be assessed. For specialized or uncommon operations, examiners tend to focus on specific points. The candidate must remain calm (and not panic) when asked about these rare operations because it is not the technical details that the examiners want to hear, but rather they would like to assess the candidate's understanding of the basic principles.

Standard operations

If you are asked about a standard operation, then it is best to provide a clear answer emphasizing three key points in the allocated time. For these types of questions, it is important to communicate the operative steps. The discussion begins in the preoperative period by confirming the diagnosis, obtaining informed consent and marking the patient. Safety and the avoidance of complications are key. When possible, describe the operation in terms of relevant anatomy. Avoid prolonged narratives of minor steps. The operative steps should be described in a way indicating your personal surgical experience and not from an operative textbook. For example, if you are asked to perform anterior cervical decompression and fusion (ACDF) then it is expected that you will describe the whole procedure from start to finish in the allocated time. No prompting should be required. Please ensure that you localize the correct level, avoid injury to the surrounding structures (pharynx/oesophagus/trachea/recurrent laryngeal nerve injury), and be certain that the posterior longitudinal ligament is opened.

Complex operations

If you are asked about a complex operation, then it is best to start the discussion with the required preoperative investigations, alternative treatments, surgical indications, and obtaining informed consent (with the benefits and risks of surgery). If you are specifically asked to describe the steps of the operation, you may wish to mention briefly that you do not have personal experience in performing it. It is important to discuss the key salient features and that you would involve the multidisciplinary team (MDT), when appropriate. The reason for these questions is to test your neuroanatomy knowledge and to see if you are aware of potential complications leading to post-operative morbidity.

For example, if you are asked to debulk a pineal tumour, it is important to confirm the diagnosis with the appropriate radiological imaging and evaluate serum and cerebrospinal fluid (CSF) tumour markers. Indicate the management if hydrocephalus is present. Treatment includes close observation while awaiting surgery, external ventricular drainage (EVD), endoscopic third ventriculostomy (ETV) ± biopsy or insertion of a ventricular peritoneal (VP) shunt. When asked to describe the operative steps, mention anatomical landmarks and key safety points. Mention the common approaches (infratentorial supracerebellar, occipital transtentorial and transcallosal interhemispheric), preservation of the deep venous system (internal cerebral veins, vein of Galen and basal vein of Rosenthal), and avoidance of a complete tumour resection if the midbrain tectum is grossly infiltrated.

In summation, this is analogous to general surgery operations. On the one hand, if asked to describe how to do an appendicectomy, then the examiner wants to know all the operative steps. On the other hand, if asked how to perform a Whipple's procedure, then the examiner wants to know the general principles, key anatomical steps and overall management (e.g. coagulopathy, total parenteral nutrition and percutaneous transhepatic cholangiography and drainage as a temporary measure).

Moreover, it is important to familiarize yourself with the 'tools' used during neurosurgical operations. Key topics include CUSA (cavitron ultrasonic surgical aspirator), microscopic-integrated ICG (IndoCyanine Green), high-speed drills, neuronavigation and 5-ALA (5-aminolevulinic acid) fluorescence-guided surgery.

In this section of the examination, the examiner assesses your surgical anatomy, knowledge and how you avoid potential surgical complications. Therefore, it must be stressed that for the operative surgery viva, the main emphasis is on surgical anatomy of the approach and complication avoidance.

Anatomical landmarks

With emphasis on neuroanatomy, the cranio-cerebral relationships are frequently asked. The following are key favourite anatomical landmarks.

Central sulcus

The central sulcus is an anatomical landmark along a straight line from a point midway between the lateral canthus and ear canal (or from a point about 5 cm straight up from the ear canal) to a point about 2 cm posterior to the mid-distance between the nasion and inion in the midline. This makes the motor cortex more or less in line with the ear canal near the midline or about 4–5 cm posterior to the coronal suture.

Calcarine fissure

The calcarine fissure is an anatomical landmark located at the caudal end of the medial surface of the brain. The calcarine sulcus begins near the occipital pole in two converging rami and runs forward to a point a little below the splenium of the corpus callosum, where it is joined at an acute angle by the medial part of the parieto-occipital sulcus. The anterior part of this fissure gives rise to the prominence of the calcar avis in the posterior cornu of the lateral ventricle.

Foramen of Monro

The foramen of Monro connects the paired lateral ventricles with the third ventricle at the midline of the brain. The trajectory to the foramen is in line with the coronal suture (as it meets the superior temporal line).

Lateral limb of the Sylvian fissure

The lateral limb of the Sylvian fissure lies along a line connecting the lateral canthus to three-quarters the distance between the nasion and inion in the midline.

Parieto-occipital sulcus

The lateral part of the sulcus is situated about 5 cm in front of the occipital pole. The medial part runs downward and forward as a deep cleft on the medial surface of the hemisphere, and joins the calcarine fissure below and behind the posterior end of the corpus callosum. In most cases it contains a submerged gyrus. It marks the boundary between the cuneus and precuneus, and also between the parietal and occipital lobes. It is located approximately in line with the lambdoid suture.

Transverse sinus

The transverse sinuses are of large size and begin at the internal occipital protuberance; one, generally the right, being the direct continuation of the superior sagittal sinus, the other the continuation of the straight sinus. They drain from the confluence of sinuses to the sigmoid sinuses, which ultimately connect to the internal jugular vein.

Further examples of important intracranial landmarks

Anterior ethmoidal foramen

The anterior ethmoidal foramen is a small opening formed when the anterior ethmoidal notch on the superior margin of the ethmoid bone corresponds to a similar small notch in the frontal bone creating a small foramen in the sutural junction of the two bones. The foramen transmits the anterior ethmoidal nerve, a branch of the nasociliary nerve, into the anterior and middle ethmoidal sinuses and nasal cavity. It also indicates the anterior extent of the cribriform plate. Identification of the anterior ethmoidal artery is an important landmark in endonasal endoscopic surgery as it passes from the orbit to anterior cranial fossa.

Arcuate eminence

This is a distinct, rounded prominence on the superior surface of the petrous temporal bone. It sits about halfway between the petrosquamous suture and the apex of the bone. This rounded eminence marks the position of the anterior semicircular canal in the inner ear.

First denticulate ligament

The denticulate ligament is located in the pia mater of the spinal cord. It attaches the pia mater to the arachnoid and dura maters. The first ligament separates the spinal accessory nerve (which is the only motor root that is dorsal to the denticulate ligaments) from the vertebral artery.

Flocculus

The flocculus is the smallest lobe of the cerebellum. It is located at the anterior part of the hemisphere, between the biventral lobe and the middle peduncle of the cerebellum, in the line of the horizontal fissure. Boundaries: inferior to cranial nerves VII/VIII and superior to cranial nerves IX/X/XI.

Frontal horn of the lateral ventricle

The frontal horn is a portion of the lateral ventricle that passes forward and laterally, from the interventricular foramen into the frontal lobe, curving around the anterior end of the caudate nucleus. Its floor is formed by the upper surface of the reflected portion of the corpus callosum, the rostrum. It is bounded medially by the anterior portion of the septum pellucidum, and laterally by the head of the caudate nucleus. Its apex reaches the posterior surface of the genu of the corpus callosum. It is located deep to the inferior frontal gyrus.

Temporal horn of the lateral ventricle

The temporal horn traverses the temporal lobe of the brain, forming in its course a curve around the posterior end of the thalamus. Its floor is composed of the hippocampus, the fimbria hippocampi, the collateral eminence, and the choroid plexus. Its roof is formed chiefly by the inferior surface of the tapetum of the corpus callosum, but the tail of the caudate nucleus and the stria terminalis also extend forward in the roof of the inferior cornu to its extremity; the tail of the caudate nucleus joins the putamen. It is located deep to the middle temporal gyrus.

Lateral mesencephalic sulcus

At this sulcus, cranial nerve IV disappears inferior to the tentorial edge.

Limen insulae

The limen insulae forms the junction point between the anterior and posterior stem of the Sylvian fissure. It is the most lateral limit of the anterior perforated substance and the starting point of the insular cortex. It has a close relationship to the middle cerebral artery (MCA) and branches.

Operative surgery and surgical anatomy

Introduction to operative surgery

1. Obtain informed consent from the patient, explaining the risks and benefits of the surgical procedure.
2. Ensure the appropriate side is marked.
3. Ensure radiological imaging and equipment is checked.
4. Note that the procedure will be performed with the patient under general anaesthetic, with a urinary catheter in place and preoperative antibiotics and steroids provided at the time of induction (if appropriate).
5. Note positioning of the patient.
6. Ensure standard preparation and drape.

Case 1

A 35-year-old man presents with a World Federation of Neurological Societies (WFNS) Grade II subarachnoid haemorrhage (SAH) secondary to anterior circulation aneurysm. His aneurysm is not suitable for endovascular coiling. He has been scheduled for surgery.

Pterional craniotomy

- General anaesthetic is employed.
- IV antibiotics are begun.
- The patient is placed in the supine position with head elevated and rotated away from the operative side (ensuring the malar eminence is the highest point in the surgical field).
- A pterional incision begins superiorly on the midline at the anterior edge of the hairline (e.g. at the widow's peak) and extended inferiorly (remaining behind the hairline) to within 1 cm of the superior aspect of the zygoma, 1 cm anterior to the external auditory canal.
- Skin and myocutaneous flap are reflected in one layer.
- A burr hole is place in the keyhole position while ensuring the orbit is protected.
- Another burr hole is placed just above the zygoma.
- A free bone flap is fashioned.
- The inner table of frontal bone and greater and lesser wing of the sphenoid are drilled until flush with the anterior cranial fossa floor.
- Dura is opened in a semicircular fashion.
- A brain spatula is used to retract the frontal lobe and to release CSF from the optico-carotid cistern.

Case 2

A 22-year-old man presents with headaches and blurred vision. His magnetic resonance imaging (MRI) scan demonstrates a colloid cyst in the anterior third ventricle. He has been scheduled for surgery.

Transcallosal approach

- General anaesthetic is employed.
- IV antibiotics are begun.
- The patient is in a supine position with the head in a neutral position (Mayfield 3-point pin fixation).
- The head is elevated to 30°.
- A curved skin incision is made over the coronal suture.
  - Approximately two-thirds anterior and one-third posterior to the coronal suture.
- 2 burr holes are placed on the superior sagittal sinus.
- Free bone flap is fashioned with 1 cm on the left and 3 cm on the right side. The craniotomy is about 6 cm in length and 5 cm in width.
- Budde halo retractor system is assembled.
- U-shaped dural flap is made. A curved durotomy is made with the base over the superior sagittal sinus. The dural edge is then secured and hitched.
- Arachnoid granulation is dissected free from the base.
- Care is taken not to sacrifice the cortical veins.
- Using a hand-held retractor, gentle retraction is placed along the interhemispheric fissure.
- Identify the following structures:
  - Callasomarginal and pericallosal arteries.
  - Cingulate gyrus.
  - Pericallosal arteries.
  - Corpus callosum (pearly white colour).
- When both pericallosal arteries are identified, the callosal section of <2 cm is made between the two arteries (avoid the penetrating branches).
- The cauterized ependymal layer is opened for entry into the lateral ventricles.
- The orientation of the ventricle is confirmed by the configuration of the choroid plexus and thalamostriate vein, which courses anteriorly in a medial direction to reach the foramen of Monro.
- Foraminal entry via the foramen of Monro, especially if it has been dilated by the presence of hydrocephalus, is the least traumatic. The choroidal fissure can be opened posteriorly to enlarge the foramen of Monro.
- If the lesion is not accessible via foraminal entry, the interforniceal approach is utilized. The interforniceal approach is achieved by a callosotomy that is as close as possible to the midline.
- A colloid cyst wall is firm, smooth and greyish in colour. Attachment of cyst at tela choroidae is identified and released.

Transcallosal resection of colloid cyst

Key points and safety considerations

Position head and location of craniotomy – note location of burr holes.

Avoid compression of superior sagittal sinus (SSS) by medial retractor (if used).

Take care to avoid damage of supplementary motor cortex by retraction or cingulate gyrus by misidentifying the callosomarginal artery as pericallosal artery.

Perform septum pellucidotomy.

Take care in handling the fornix.

Insert an EVD for safety to prevent post-operative hydrocephalus from intraventricular haemorrhage.

Potential pitfalls

Anatomical landmarks – do not just rely on image guidance because the coronal suture is in line with the foramen of Monro in the true coronal plane,

If cyst is located in the posterior third ventricular roof, it is better to choose a subforniceal transchoroidal approach via taenia fornices rather than divide the fornix.

Identify the correct foramen of Monro (lateralization).

Case 3

A 57-year-old woman presents with headaches, facial pain and an unsteady gait. Her MRI scan demonstrates a petroclival tumour. She has been scheduled for surgery.

Subtemporal transtentorial approach

- General anaesthetic is employed.
- IV antibiotics are begun.
- The patient is placed in a lateral position.
- The head is elevated to 30°.
- Skin incision: a reverse horseshoe skin incision is made starting from the zygoma 1 cm anterior to the tragus, extending above the pinna and curving down about 2 cm behind the mastoid.
- The scalp flap is reflected inferiorly down the zygoma. Care is taken not to enter the external auditory canal.
- Burr hole is made in the squamous portion of the temporal lobe immediately above the roof of the zygoma.
- A temporal craniotomy is made with its posterior extent just above the mastoid, and additional bone is removed down to the middle fossa floor.
- Mastoid air cells are waxed.
- Extradural dissection is performed from a lateral-to-medial and posterior-to-anterior direction to avoid stretching the greater superficial petrosal nerve (GSPN) branch of the facial nerve.
- The following landmarks are identified: tegmen tympani, arcuate eminence, lesser superficial petrosal nerve (LSPN), GSPN, middle meningeal artery, and mandibular branch of the trigeminal nerve. The LSPN can be distinguished from the GSPN by its joining with the middle meningeal artery at the foramen spinosum.
- The dura is opened with a T-shaped incision along the inferior temporal lobe and with a vertical limb along the middle fossa floor.
- Retraction of the temporal lobe is performed with the aid the microscope.
- Temporal lobe elevation is limited by vein of Labbé.
- Cranial nerve IV is identified; the division of the tentorium begins immediately posterior, near the petrous ridge. The tentorial division is extended 3–4 cm posterolaterally and a couple of millimetres posterior to the superior petrosal sinus without injuring the sigmoid sinus. The division of the tentorium is carried in an anterolateral direction into the middle fossa and across the superior petrosal sinus with ligatures or clips. This results in a triangular flap with a view down onto the clivus.

Subtemporal approach

Key points and safety considerations

Consider a lumbar drain (if no contraindication, e.g. a large mass). CSF retrieval from cisterns requires retraction.

Preserve vein of Labbé.

Be aware of the location of cranial nerve IV at tentorial hiatus.

Potential pitfalls

Anatomy of vein of Labbé and variations in number and configuration

Case 4

A 63-year-old woman presents with progressive visual loss and ophthalmoplegia. Her MRI scan demonstrates a pituitary macroadeoma. Her pituitary function tests (including prolactin) are normal. She has been scheduled for surgery.

Transsphenoidal approach

- General anaesthetic is employed.
- IV antibiotics are begun.
- The patient is placed in a supine position with the head in a neutral position resting on a donut.
- Equipment: image intensifier and microscope are in place.
- The lateral thigh is prepared.
- 0.25% xylocaine and adrenaline infiltrated into the nasal mucosa.
- Octrivine nasal spray is used to reduce nasal congestion.
- Apply adequate aqueous-based antiseptic solution.
- The operative surgeon stands at the cranial end of the operative table or on the right side of the patient.
- Right-sided transnasal paraseptal approach is used.
- A curved incision is made along in the mucosa-cutaneous junction along the columella or deep over the bony/cartilaginous junction of the nasal septum, e.g. Kellihan.
- Sub-perichondral dissection is performed.
- A long hand-held nasal speculum (e.g. Kellihan) is used to advance and fracture the perpendicular plate of the ethmoid bone.
- Orientation along the sagittal plane is checked regularly with fluoroscopy.
- Identify the sphenoid ostium and keel of the rostrum.
- Anterior wall of sphenoid sinus is entered using an osteotome or drill.
- The opening may be widened with Kerrison rongeurs.
- Septation within the sphenoid sinus is identified on a CT scan.
- Cruciate durotomy is made.
- Use angled ring curettes, tumour forceps and suction to gently debulk the tumour.
- Apply a Valsalva manoeuvre to deliver the remaining tumour.

Complications of the transsphenoidal approach

- Epistaxis.
- Nasal perforation.
- Sinusitis.
- Visual impairment (ophthalmoplegia and loss of vision).
- Transient/permanent diabetes insipidus.
- CSF rhinorrhea.
- Meningitis.
- Damage to surrounding structures (cavernous sinus, intracavernous cranial nerves and carotid artery).

Transsphenoidal resection of pituitary adenoma

Key points and safety considerations

Consider image guidance in cases that are re-do or extended approaches or have difficult sellar anatomy when performing endoscopic or microscopic-assisted transsphenoidal surgery.

Avoid carotid injury – identify the 'kissing' carotids, avoid avulsion of a laterally placed intrasphenoid sinus septum inserting into the carotid canal, and carefully identify anatomical landmarks and midline when drilling.

The order of resection of large macroadenomas is to avoid premature descent of the diaphragm sellae.

For endoscopic cases, different angled scopes are used to inspect the sella for complete surgical resection.

Potential pitfalls

Be aware of true invasion of cavernous sinus vs. compression.

Be aware of the need for total resection for secretory vs. nonsecretory adenomas.

Case 5

A 24-year-old man presents with headache, visual deterioration and vomiting. His MRI scan demonstrated non-communicating (obstructive) hydrocephalus secondary to aqueductal stenosis. He has been scheduled for surgery.

Endoscopic third ventriculostomy (ETV)

- General anaesthetic is employed.
- IV antibiotics are begun.
- The patient is placed in a supine position with the patient's head in a neutral position on a horseshoe headrest.
- The head is then elevated to minimize excessive CSF loss and air entry.
- A linear, S- or U-curved shaped skin incision is made.
- A burr hole is placed 3 cm lateral to the midline and 1 cm anterior to the coronal suture.
- A cruciate durotomy is made.
- No. 14 French peel-away catheter is then used to cannulate the lateral ventricle.
- The stylet is removed to ensure the placement into the ventricular system.
- The two leaves are peeled away and stapled to the drapes.
- A rigid endoscope is passed through the sheath and the lateral ventricle is visualized.
- Important structures to identify are foramen of Monro, choroid plexus and thamalostriate veins.
- The scope is advanced further through the foramen into the third ventricle.
- The landmarks located on the floor of the third ventricle are the following:
  - Mammillary bodies posteriorly.
  - Infundibular recess anteriorly.
  - Thin, transparent floor of the third ventricle.
  - Basilar artery visualized through the thinned floor.
- No. 4 French Fogarty balloon catheter is advanced through the opening into the floor, 0.2 mL of fluid is instilled into the balloon and the balloon is inflated to widen the newly created aperture.
- After advancing the endoscope into the prepontine cistern, the arachnoid bands are released.
- Inspect for cerebrospinal fluid flow through the fenestration.
- Consider insertion of an external ventricular drain if the patient was previously shunt dependent or very symptomatic preoperatively or if the procedure was complicated by bleeding.

Endoscopic third ventriculostomy (ETV)

Key points and safety considerations

Position of burr hole and trajectory.

Anatomical landmarks.

Location and performance of stoma to avoid stretching or damage of basilar artery or P1 perforators.

Anatomical attachment of second membrane/ medial extension of Lilliquist's membrane.

Potential pitfalls

Do not proceed without adequate visualisation of anatomical landmarks.

If an endoscopic biopsy of an intracranial lesion is also required, perform ETV first because bleeding from the biopsy site may obscure the view and preclude completion of the ETV.

Case 6

A 32-year-old woman presents with a chronic history of neck pain and intermittent suboccipital headaches that are worse with neck extension and coughing. Her MRI scan demonstrated a Chiari malformation type I with no evidence of hydrocephalus. She has been scheduled for surgery.

Foramen magnum decompression

- General anaesthetic is employed.
- IV antibiotics are begun.
- Procedure is performed in prone position with head secured on Mayfield 3-point pin skull clamp.
- The patient's neck is placed in 'marching army position' (neck extended and flexed at the atlanto-occipital junction).
- Ensure no venous congestion.
- Linear midline incision is made extending from the level of inion (external occipital protuberance) to C2 spinous process.
- Bilateral paraspinous muscles are stripped with monopolar diathermy.
- Subperiosteal dissection over C1, C2 and occiput is performed.
- Identify the C2 spinous process and the inion.

- Four burr holes are made and connected by using a craniotome. The bone flap is then elevated.
- The posterior arch of C1 may need to be removed.
- Ensure adequate haematosis.
- Careful Y-shaped durotomy is made while keeping the arachnoid layer intact.

Foramen magnum decompression

Key points and safety considerations

Ensure correct indications for surgery, differentiate between those with or without syrinx and look for significant anterior additional pathology.

Avoid overflexion while positioning (± somatosensory evoked potentials [SSEPs]).

Tailor bone decompression.

Protect tonsillar loops of posterior inferior cerebellar artery (PICA).

Consider checking CSF flow at end of procedure with ultrasound guidance.

Potential pitfalls

Describe same procedure regardless of presentation and anatomical variation.

Be able to debate reasons for chosen technique (e.g. opening dura ± opening arachnoid).

Case 7

A 54-year-old man presents with craniocervical pain associated with numbness and tingling of the fingers. On clinical examination, there was evidence of long tract signs (spasticity, hyperreflexia). His MRI scan demonstrated intradural foramen magnum tumour. He has been scheduled for surgery.

Far lateral approach to the skull base

- General anaesthetic is employed.
- IV antibiotics are begun.
- The patient is placed in a park bench position with head secured on Mayfield 3-point pin skull clamp.
- Check the following:
  - Ensure no venous congestion.
  - The pressure areas are protected.
  - Equipment, radiological imaging and microscope are checked preoperatively.
- A retromastoid 'inverted hockey stick' incision is performed with the lateral limb extending below the mastoid process and the medial limb just below C3, if the lesion is below the foramen magnum.
  - Identify the superior nuchal line and follow the midline (C3 level).
- Sub-periosteal dissection of the paraspinous muscles is performed down to the level C2 and C3 spinous processes..
- Occipital bone is exposed.
- Myocutaneous flap is created and retracted infero-laterally.
- Lateral mass of C1 and vertebral artery are exposed. Vertebral artery is identified entering the dura just above C1 arch at the vertebral notch.
- Venous bleeding is controlled with diathermy.
- Depending on the size, position and type of lesion, the suboccipital craniotomy is extended to include the lateral condyle and rim of foramen magnum.
- The dura is opened in a curvilinear fashion or with three lateral triangular leaves based on the transverse sinus, sigmoid sinus and vertebral artery.

Case 8

A 45-year-old woman presents with unilateral hearing loss, tinnitus and unsteady gait. Her MRI scan demonstrated a vestibular schwannoma centred on the internal acoustic meatus (IAM). She has been scheduled for surgery.

Retrosigmoid approach

- General anaesthetic is employed.
- IV antibiotics are begun.
- The patient is placed in the park bench position.
- Ensure
  - no venous congestion.
  - facial monitoring application.
  - insertion of a lumbar drain and urinary catheter.
  - pressure areas are protected.
- Bony landmarks – mastoid process and external occipital protuberance are identified.
- Pathway of transverse sinus is identified.
- A postauricular curvilinear incision is made 2 cm behind the mastoid tip extending cephalad above the transverse sinus and caudal to include the mastoid tip.
- The muscles are reflected away by the use of diathermy. A cuff of periosteum is maintained to assist with dual closure at the end of the operation.
- Check the landmarks: asterion and mastoid.
- A burr hole is made at the asterion.
- A craniectomy is performed until both sigmoid sinus and transverse sinus are visible and inferiorly until the foramen magnum is palpable.
- Exposed mastoid air cells are occluded with bone wax.
- If there is bleeding from the mastoid emissary vein entering the transverse and sigmoid sinus, this may be controlled with Gelfoam and patties.
- Budde halo retractor is assembled.
- Cruciate durotomy is performed to the junction of transverse and sigmoid sinus.
- The cerebellum is relaxed by releasing CSF from arachnoid.
- A narrow 3-mm brain spatula is introduced parallel and below the superior petrosal sinus.

Retrosigmoid craniotomy

Key points and safety considerations

Landmarks of transverse and sigmoid sinuses – mastoid and digastric groove.

CSF retrieval from the cisterna magna.

Avoidance of excessive cerebellar retraction.

Correct identification of cranial nerves – landmarks.

Potential pitfalls

Knowledge of neurophysiological cranial nerve monitoring.

'Pros and cons' of preservation of vein of Dandy.

Case 9

A 66-year-old man presents with progressive bilateral hand weakness, in that he is now dropping objects. His cervical MRI scan demonstrated cervical spondylosis with spinal cord compression. He has been scheduled for surgery.

Anterior cervical discectomy and fusion (ACDF)

- General anaesthetic is employed.
- IV antibiotics are begun.
- The patient is placed in a supine position with the neck slightly extended.
- A right-sided approach is used.
- Linear skin incision is made along Langer's line. Placement of this incision is important.
- Exposure is performed in layers.
- Platysma is cut and undermined.
- The investing layer of cervical fascia is divided along the anterior border of sternocleidomastoid (SCM) to define the plane between the carotid sheath laterally and the larynx, trachea and oesophagus medially.
- A combination of a careful sharp and blunt dissection is used, initially medial to SCM and lateral to superior belly of omohyoid.
- At this stage it is essential to palpate for the carotid artery and continue medially to the carotid artery toward the spine. A handheld Cloward retractor is used.
- Blunt dissection of prevertebral fascia using peanut sponges is used to expose both longus colli muscles.
- The level is confirmed with X-ray. Use a spinal needle in the disc space as a marker to identify the correct level.
- Once this is achieved, Cloward's or black-belt retractors are inserted underneath the medial border of both longus colli muscles.
- A box shaped incision is made over the anterior longitudinal ligament (ALL) and extended laterally to the uncal-vertebral joint. The anterior annulus is incised.
- Using a microscope, the disc fragments are removed using rongeurs and curettes.
- A high-speed drill is used to gentle burr the bony endplates and to remove osteophytes and the posterior uncinate process.
- The dissection is continued laterally until the upslope of the uncinate process is encountered.
- Once the posterior osteophyte is removed with a high-speed drill, the posterior longitudinal ligament is removed using a 1-mm Kerrison rongeur.
- Careful exploration with a blunt hook probe alongside the nerve root confirms adequate compression.
- A trial cage is inserted under X-ray guidance.
- The cage (with bone graft) is gently tapped into place with a hammer and mallet.
- An anterior cervical plate may be placed at this point.
- Haemostasis is achieved.
- A gravity drain is inserted.

Complications of ACDF

- Infection.
- Bleeding (including haematoma).
- CSF leakage.
- Recurrence.
- Failure.
- Further surgery.
- Progression.
- Paralysis (nerve root or spinal cord injury).
- Hoarse voice (recurrent laryngeal injury).
- Hypoglossal nerve or superior laryngeal nerve injury.
- Swallowing difficulties.
- Pneumothorax.
- Oesophageal perforation.
- Carotid artery injury.
- Horner's syndrome.
- Pseudoarthrosis.
- Instability.
- Instrumentation failure.

Case 10

A 33-year-old man presents with back pain coupled with right leg pain radiating into his sole, coupled with a foot drop. His lumbar MRI scan demonstrated a large right-sided L4/5 lumbar disc protrusion. He has been scheduled for surgery.

Lumbar microdiscectomy

- General anaesthetic is employed.
- IV antibiotics are begun.
- The patient is placed in a prone position on a Wilson frame or Montreal mattress.
- Preoperative X-ray is used to confirm the correct level.
- Surgery is conducted from the ipsilateral to the symptomatic side.
- A midline linear skin incision is performed.
- Exposure is performed in layers.
- Subperiosteal paraspinous muscle dissection is achieved with monopolar diathermy.
- The interspace is identified.
- A foraminotomy is performed using a mixture of Kerrison punches and rongeurs.
- Medial aspect of the facet is removed.
- The bone edges are waxed to achieve haemostasis.
- With the assistance of the operative microscope, ligamentum flavum is excised using sharp and blunt dissection. Bipolar coagulation of epidural veins may be required.
- The nerve root is identified and then gently retracted/protected medially.
- If a free disc fragment is seen in the canal, it is removed with a pituitary rongeur.
- If the fragment is under the thecal sac, the fragment can be brought forward with a nerve hook.
- If the disc fragment is contained within the annulus, a further incision (rectangle or a single cut parallel to the nerve root) is made over the annulus.
- If the disc fragment is intradural, the dura will need to be opened.

Complications of lumbar microdiscectomy

- Infection.
- Bleeding (including haematoma).
- CSF leakage.
- Recurrence.
- Further surgery.
- Progression.
- Paralysis (nerve root or cauda equina injury).
- Sphincter dysfunction (bowel, urinary or sexual).
- Instability.

Overall outcome

- 70–75% of patients experience a significant improvement in their leg pain.
- 20–25% of patients improve but report persistent leg pain.
- 5% of patients have no benefit at all.
- 1% of patients deteriorate (leg pain).

Special case: Far lateral discectomy for extraforaminal disc herniation

- General anaesthetic is employed.
- IV antibiotics are begun.
- The patient is placed in a prone position on a Wilson frame or Montreal mattress.
- Preoperative X-ray is used to confirm needle placement on the correct level.
- Surgery is conducted from the ipsilateral symptomatic side.
- Standard preparation and drape is performed.
- Paramedian intertransverse approach: a linear incision 2.5 cm off the midline is made.
- Paraspinous muscles are split along the line of the fibres to expose the transverse process and facet joint.
- Intraoperative X-ray is used to confirm the correct level.
- The operative microscope is used.
- The intertransverse ligament is incised and reflected.
- Careful dissection is carried out to expose the pedicle and pars interarticularis to identify the roof of the foramen.
- The exiting nerve root can be seen underneath the pars.
- The root is then mobilized caudally to expose the prolapsed disc.

Case 11

A 31-year-old man was involved in a motorbike accident. He was thrown off his motorbike when he was hit by a moving vehicle. He presents with severe back pain radiating into the dorsum of his foot. His lumbar CT scan demonstrates an isolated lumbar burst fracture. He has been scheduled for surgery.

Lumbar pedicle screw fixation

- Preoperative planning (X-rays, CT scan ± MRI scan) for deciding the bone quality, pedicle transverse diameter and screw trajectory may be required.

- General anaesthetic is employed.
- IV antibiotics are begun.
- The patient is placed in the prone position on a Wilson frame or Montreal mattress.
- Preoperative X-ray is used to confirm the correct level.
- Midline linear skin incision is performed. Exposure performed in layers.
- Monopolar cautery is done through fascia in midline to the spinous processes.
- Bilateral subperiosteal dissection of paraspinal muscles exposes the transverse processes.
- Self-retaining retractors are inserted.

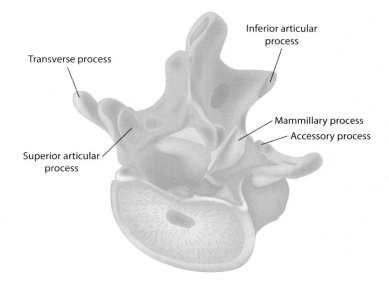

Figure 4.1 Lumbar vertebra

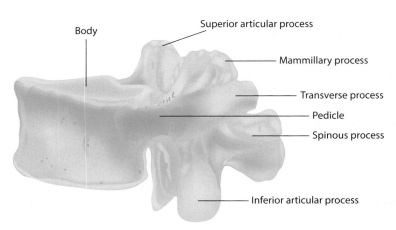

Figure 4.2 Lumbar vertebra, sagittal view

- Posterior instrumented lumbar spine fusion is performed using pedicle screws one level rostral and caudal to the fracture (extended if the fracture is at the thoracolumbar junction).

Entry point for lumbar pedicle screw

Entry point is the junction of the lateral facet and the transverse process or bisection of a vertical line through the facet joints and a horizontal line through the transverse process. The key anatomical points are the facet joint, transverse process and pars interarticularis.

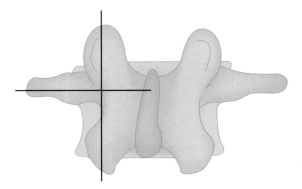

Figure 4.3 Lumbar pedicle entry point

- After decorticating the pedicle entry site with a burr and penetrating the site with an awl, a curved or straight pedicle probe is used to develop a path for the screw through the cancellous bone of the pedicle into the vertebral body.

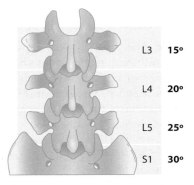

L3	15°
L4	20°
L5	25°
S1	30°

Figure 4.4 Coronal lumbar spine

- The coronal plane angle increases approximately 5° per level from L1 to sacrum.
- A pedicle feeler is inserted down the created pathway to confirm the pedicle walls are intact.
- The pedicles are then tapped.
- After cannulation and confirmation of the pedicle with the appropriate trajectory, the largest possible pedicle screw is placed (length: determined by measuring the length of the probe from the pedicle entry site to a depth of 50–80% of the vertebral body).
- The screws usually have a diameter of 4.5–7 mm, and a length of 35–50 mm.
- After pedicle screw placement, the transverse process and the lateral aspects of the facet joints are decorticated, the pedicle screws are connected to a longitudinal construct (a rod) and top locking nuts are applied.
- A bone graft is then applied along the transverse process and the construct.

Case 12

A 74-year-old man presents with impaired memory, gait disturbance and urinary incontinence. His MRI scan demonstrated communicating hydrocephalus. He will undergo lumbar infusion to investigate normal pressure hydrocephalus.

Lumbar infusion studies

- Pressure recording was calibrated stepwise between 0 and 50 mmHg.
- The initial steady-state CSF pressure was recorded (until a stable initial pressure curve for at least 10 minutes was obtained) before starting a constant rate (0.80 mL/min) infusion of Ringer's solution.
- The CSF pressure is continuously recorded through the other needle via the pressure-monitoring device connected to a printer.
- The CSF pressure is recorded continuously during a period of at least 45 minutes to establish a steady-state pressure plateau representing the pressure level at which absorption balanced infusion.
- If steady-state plateau pressure exceeds 22 mmHg, intervention (shunt insertion) is likely to be beneficial.

Case 13

An 83-year-old woman presents with severe stabbing electric facial pain in a V1 and V2 disturbance. Her MRI scan demonstrated vascular compression of the trigeminal nerve at the root entry zone. She has been scheduled for surgery (see Table 4.1).

Percutaneous trigeminal rhizotomy (PTR)

- Symptomatic side is marked.
- General anaesthetic is applied with a laryngeal mask airway.
- IV antibiotics are begun.
- The patient is placed supine in a neutral position.
- Hartel's anatomical landmark is used to guide the needle by aid of fluoroscopy.

Three anatomical landmarks are identified on the patient's face:

1. The point supero-lateral to the zygoma and 3 cm in front of the tragus.
2. The point at the intersection of the same axial plane and the midpupillary line.
3. The point 3 cm lateral to the mouth's corner on the bicommissural line.

- 5 mL of xylocaine 1% with adrenaline (epinephrine) is used as local infiltration.
- Placing your index finger inside the mouth, a 22G spinal needle is used to guide the needle toward the foramen ovale.
- X-ray guides the needle to the correct location in the trigeminal cistern.
- The foramen ovale is seen through the pterygo-mandibular and infratemporal space as an oval structure at the top of the petrous pyramid.
- The patient may wince when the needle penetrates the foramen.
- When the tip of the cannula is located inside the arachnoid of trigeminal cistern, there may be spontaneous egress of CSF.
- Iohexol is injected into the cistern as the table is tilted upward to outline Meckel's cave.
- The inferior edge of the gasserian ganglion can be seen as the superior edge of the outlined space. The amount of iohexol to fill the cistern is m____ by injecting until the dye over-flo____ ____sterior fossa. The iohexol is ____ ____drous glycerol is injected ____ the cistern.

Table 4.1 Results of surgical treatments for trig____

	Radiofrequency rhizotomy				lar ion
Total number of patients treated	5(				
Initial pain relief	9.				
Recurrence rate	20%				
Facial numbness	98%				
Anaesthesia dolorosa	0.2%				%
Corneal anaesthesia	3%				0.05%
Perioperative morbidity	0.6%				10%

Adapted from Taha JM, Tew JM. Comparison of surgical treatmen____ ____uation of radiofrequency rhizotomy. *Neurosurgery* 1996; 38(5): 865–71.

Case 14

A 34-year-old man sustains a severe head injury following a motorcycle crash. His CT scan demonstrated a diffuse subarachnoid haemorrhage and sulci effacement. He has been scheduled for surgery.

Insertion of an intracranial pressure (ICP) bolt

- General or local anaesthetic is employed.
- IV antibiotics are begun.
- The patient is placed supine with the head in a neutral position.
- Kocher's point (coronal) places the catheter in the frontal horn. If no clinical indications, select the non-dominant hemisphere (right side).
- Entry site is 2–3 cm from the midline in the mid-pupillary line and 1 cm anterior to the coronal suture.

- Open the cranial access kit and the Camino bolt in a sterile fashion.
- Stab incision is performed over the planned burr hole site.
- Place a twist drill hole through skull without penetrating the dura.
- Use the safety nut on the drill to prevent plunging.
- Screw the bolt into the skull until finger tight.
- Open the dura with a probe (available in the cranial access kit).
- Direct the catheter perpendicular to the brain's surface to a depth of 5–7 cm.
- Confirm a waveform is present.
- Tighten the bolt around the catheter to secure in place.

Case 15

A 55-year-old woman presents with a sudden-onset severe headache, vomiting and photophobia. While in the emergency department she becomes confused and drowsy, and her GCS drops. Her CT scan demonstrated an extensive subarachnoid haemorrhage with intraventricular extension. She has been scheduled for surgery.

External ventricular drainage (ventriculostomy)

- General, regional or local anaesthetic is employed.
- IV antibiotics are begun.
- The patient is placed supine with the head in a neutral position.
- Kocher's point (coronal) places the catheter in the frontal horn. If no clinical indications, select the non-dominant hemisphere (right side).
- Entry site is 2–3 cm from midline in the mid-pupillary line and 1 cm anterior to the coronal suture.
- A burr hole is created by holding the perforator perpendicular to the skull.
- Dura is opened.

- Bipolar cautery is used to coagulate the dural edges.
- A ventricular catheter is inserted perpendicular to the brain surface to a depth of 5–6 cm and aimed toward the ipsilateral medial canthus.
- The stylet is withdrawn from the catheter to check for CSF flow.
- The opening pressure is measured.
- A tunnelling device is attached to the distal end of the catheter. Stabilize the catheter at the burr hole and tunnel the distal portion under the galea aponeurosis to a skin exit site at least 5 cm away from the entry point.
- Reconfirm CSF drainage.
- Close the galea aponeurosis with 2.0 Vicryl and apply skin clips.
- The catheter is secured to the scalp with a U stitch with 3.0 nylon.
- The distal end of the catheter is connected to a drainage system.

Post-operative considerations

- Send CSF for analysis (biochemistry, bacteriology ± cytology).

Case 16

A 28-year-old woman presents with headaches, vomiting and abducens palsy. On fundoscopy, there is evidence of papilloedema. Her CT scan demonstrated hydrocephalus with periventricular lucency. She has been scheduled for surgery.

Ventriculoperitoneal (VP) shunt insertion

- General anaesthetic is employed.
- IV antibiotics are begun.
- The patient is placed supine with the head turned 90° to the opposite side with ipsilateral shoulder roll in place.
- Shunt is assembled.
- If no specific clinical indications, select the non-dominant hemisphere (right side) as the entry site. Scalp incision is a small semilunar scalp flap or linear incision.

    Frontal approach: Kocher's point (coronal) places the catheter in the frontal horn. Entry site: 2–3 cm from the midline in the mid-pupillary line and 1 cm anterior to the coronal suture.

    Occipital-parietal approach: Frazier burr hole: 3–4 cm from the midline, 6–7 cm above the inion.

    Parietal boss: flat portion of the parietal bone. 3 cm above and 3 cm posterior to the top of the pinna.

    Abdominal approach: Create a horizontal incision, 2 cm lateral and 2 cm superior to the umbilicus. The anterior rectus sheath is incised. Rectus muscle is split in layers. Long clamps are placed on posterior rectus sheath and then incised. Additional clamps are placed on the peritoneum.

- Burr hole:

    Retractors pulled caudally in order for the burr hole to be placed 1 cm below the incision to ensure that no hardware lies under the suture line. The burr hole is created by holding the perforator perpendicular to the skull.

- Dural opening:

    Bipolar cautery is used to coagulate the dural edges.

- Tunnel the shunt from the scalp to the abdominal incision by inserting a metal trocar/passer in which the shunt is then passed.
- Cannulate the ventricles. The ventricular catheter is inserted perpendicular to the brain surface.

    Frontal approach: The catheter is inserted to a depth of 5–6 cm. Aim towards the ipsilateral medial canthus.

    Occipital-parietal approach: The catheter is inserted to a depth of 3 cm.

    The stylet is withdrawn from the catheter to ensure CSF flow and to measure the opening pressure.

- Assemble the shunt.
- Connect the value between proximal and distal catheter. Secure with a silk tie.
- Assess catheter placement.
    - Check for spontaneous CSF flow from distal end.
    - 10 mL of CSF is gently aspirated from the distal catheter with a blunt needle.
    - The shunt value is easily pumped.
- Place peritoneal catheter.
    - The shunt is placed in the perineum with non-tooth forceps.
- Close the wound.
    - Ventricular end: close galea aponeurosis with 2.0 Vicryl and then apply skin clips.
    - Distal end: close the peritoneum with 2-0 Ethicon (purse–string suture). Apply interrupted Vicryl sutures to the fascia and subcutaneous tissue, and then apply skin clips.

Post-operative considerations

- Send CSF for analysis (biochemistry, bacteriology ± cytology).
- Perform neurological observations.
- Allow the patient to eat when bowel sounds are noted (due to a paralytic ileus).
- Obtain a shunt series (AP and lateral skull, chest/abdominal X-rays).

Additional notes

- A valve is a mechanical device that regulates pressure or restricts flow. A valve typically functions as follows: when the difference between the inlet pressure and the outlet pressure exceeds the opening threshold, the valve opens.

- Designs include the following:
  - Silicone rubber mitre valve.
  - Silicone rubber slit valve.
  - Rubber diaphragm valve.
  - Metallic spring ball valve.
- The opening pressure can be low, medium or high, which corresponds to 5, 10, and 15 mm Hg, respectively.
- Anti-siphon device is a mobile membrane that narrows an orifice in response to a negative pressure. When a patient stands, there can be a siphon effect.
- Requirements of an ideal shunt are the following:
  - The resistance of an open shunt should be taken together with the natural CSF.
  - Outflow resistance (usually increased in hydrocephalus) should be close to the normal resistance to CSF outflow, i.e. $6-10$ mmHg mL^{-1} min^{-1}.
  - Flow should remain constant under constant pressure conditions.
  - Flow through the shunt should not depend on the body posture or be affected by body temperature, external (environmental) pressure (within the physiological range for subcutaneous pressure) or the pulsatile component of CSF pressure.
  - Opening and closing pressures (the pressure at which flow starts and ceases) should remain constant under the conditions listed previously.
- Reversal of flow through the shunt should be impossible.

Special cases: Craniotomies to debulk underlying space-occupying lesions (meningiomas)

Case 17

A 45-year-old woman presents with headaches. Her MRI scan demonstrated a homogeneous densely enhancing mass with a broad base of attachment along the dural border with a 'dural tail'. There is evidence of mass effect. She has been scheduled for surgery.

Convexity meningioma

- General anaesthetic is employed.
- IV antibiotics are begun.
- Preoperative steroids and antibiotics are given and a urinary catheter is inserted.
- The patient is placed supine with the head fixed on a Mayfield 3-point pin headrest.
- The head is rotated to the contralateral side to allow easy access to the tumour. The head is positioned so the bone flap overlying the tumour is parallel to the floor and elevated approximately 30°.
- When using the image guidance system, the tumour may be identified and marked on the patient's scalp.
- A curve scalp incision is used based on the location and size of tumour.
- The temporalis muscle is incised and elevated.
- A free bone flap is created using a high-speed drill.
- The dura is opened in a circular fashion based on tumour, location and size.

- The aim of excision of a convexity meningioma is to achieve complete macroscopic resection of the tumour, including the dural and bony attachments. This may necessitate taking a margin of dura of approximately 1 cm surrounding the tumour.
- The tumour is devascularized by isolating the blood supply and performing an internal debulk. This may be achieved by using the cavitron ultrasonic surgical aspirator (CUSA).
- Once you have identified the arachnoid plane, the tumour is then dissected off the surrounding brain.
- The tumour is then imploded and removed in a piecemeal fashion.
- Careful attention is paid to the arachnoid plane at the tumour–brain interface to ensure no residual tumour is left behind. Resection of the involved dura and bone may be required.
- Ensure adequate haemostasis.

Convexity meningioma

Key points and safety considerations

Location of craniotomy – image guidance.

Resection of dural tail.

Preservation of uninvolved cortical veins.

Identification of arachnoid plane and preservation of arteries.

Potential pitfalls

Drilling of a hyperostotic (meningioma infiltration) calvaria.

Defining the exact anatomical location.

Case 18

A 68-year-old woman presents with headaches, progressive unilateral visual loss and anosmia. Her MRI scan demonstrated a diffuse densely enhancing tumour arising from the anterior skull base with the anterior cerebral arteries located posterior to the lesion and the optic chiasm located inferior to the lesion. She has been scheduled for surgery.

Olfactory groove meningioma

- General anaesthetic is employed.
- IV antibiotics are begun.
- Preoperative steroids and antibiotics are given and a urinary catheter is inserted.
- The patient is placed supine with the head fixed on a Mayfield 3-point pin headrest.
- The head is neutral with 20° neck extension for subfrontal approach; the head is rotated 30° contralaterally for pterional approach.
- Bicoronal or pterional scalp incision is used, depending on the approach.
- A square of pericranium is preserved and reflected.
- Large tumours (>3 cm) are approached by a bifrontal craniotomy, then subfrontal approach. The sagittal sinus and falx are divided anteriorly. Small tumours are approached by unilateral subfrontal or pterional approach; if midline, the right side is preferred.
- For a unilateral approach, 3 burr holes are made.
  - 1 in the midline.
  - 2 laterally at the root of zygomatic process of the frontal bone.
- Care is taken not to enter the bony orbit.
- Using a high-speed drill, a free bone flap is fashioned.
- If the frontal sinus is opened the mucoperiosteum is stripped away and packed with Betadine-soaked gauze. (This will be removed at the end of the operation.)
- A 3–4 cm linear incision of the dura is made over each medial inferior frontal lobe.
- The bridging veins are coagulated and divided.

- Frontal lobe is carefully retracted laterally and posteriorly to expose the tumour.
- The tumour is devascularized by isolating the blood supply (e.g. ethmoidal arteries) at the base of the tumour.
- The tumour is internally debulked by using the CUSA.
- Once the arachnoid plane is identified, it is then dissected off the surrounding brain tissue.
- Preserve the anterior cerebral artery branches, which may be encased by the tumour.
- The tumour is then imploded and removed piecemeal.
- Careful attention is paid to the arachnoid plane at the tumour–brain interface to make sure that no residual tumour is left behind (including involved dura and bone).
- Ensure adequate haemostasis.

Olfactory groove meningioma

Key points and safety considerations

Anatomical description of olfactory groove, planum sphenoidale and tuberculum sellae.

Location and control of anterior (and posterior) ethmoidal arteries.

Limitations of techniques to preserve olfaction.

Protection of possible adherent anterior cerebral artery branches.

Decompression of optic canals if extension distally around optic nerves.

CSF repair (addressing the frontal sinus, pericranial flap, 'pros and cons' of lumbar drains).

Potential pitfalls

Attaining early control of blood supply depends largely on your chosen approach (e.g. transbasal approach).

If describing techniques such as extended endoscopic endonasal or supracilliary minicraniotomy techniques, make sure that the given lesion is suitable for such an approach and be prepared to demonstrate awareness of their difficulties and limitations

Case 19

A 58-year-old woman presents with a chronic history of headaches and now reports an unsteady gait. Her MRI scan demonstrated a frontotemporal dural-based tumour with the lesion abutting the Sylvian fissure with local mass effect. She has been scheduled for surgery.

Sphenoid wing meningioma

- Preoperative angiogram with embolization may be required.
- General anaesthetic is employed.
- IV antibiotics are begun.
- Preoperative steroids and antibiotics are given and an urinary catheter is inserted.
- The patient is placed supine with the head rotated to 30–45° degrees to the opposite side and secured in a Mayfield 3-point pin headrest.
- Mild extension (15–30°) aids in temporal lobe retraction.
- Fronto-temporal curvilinear skin incision is made extending 1 cm anterior to the tragus to 1 cm behind the hairline.
- Skin and myocutaneous flap are reflected in one layer.
- A burr hole is place in the keyhole region. Ensure the orbit is not entered.
- Another burr hole is placed just above the zygoma.
- A free bone flap is fashioned.
- A Budde halo is then assembled.
- Using a high-speed drill, the hyperostosis of greater wing of the sphenoid is drilled until flush with the middle cranial fossa floor.
- The dura is opened in a curvilinear fashion (leaving a cuff wide enough to wall off epidural bleeding and aid in dural closure), reflected and tacked with sutures.
- The tumour is devascularized by isolating the blood supply and performing an internal debulk by using the CUSA.
- Once the arachnoid plane is identified, the tumour is then dissected away from the surrounding brain tissue.
- Pay particular attention to the opercular segment of the MCA, anterior clinoid artery, carotid artery, optic nerve and the cavernous sinus.
- The area is covered with cottonoids.
- The tumour is then imploded and removed in piecemeal.
- Careful attention is paid to the arachnoid plane at the tumour–brain interface to make sure that no residual tumour is left behind (including dura and bone).
- Ensure adequate haemostasis.

Case 20

A 56-year-old woman presents with headaches, dizziness and new onset of seizures. Her MRI scan demonstrates a parafalcine dural-based lesion in the parietal lobe. She has been scheduled for surgery.

Parafalcine meningioma

- Preoperative angiogram with embolization may be required.
- General anaesthetic is employed.
- IV antibiotics are begun.
- Preoperative steroids and antibiotics are given and a urinary catheter is inserted.
- The patient is placed supine with the head fixed on a Mayfield 3-point pin headrest.
- The head is then elevated to approximately 30°.
- When using the image guidance system, the tumour may be identified and marked on the patient's scalp.
- A large reversed U-shaped flap is used. (Incorporate an additional 1 cm margin from the tumour edge.)
- Several burr holes are made over the superior sagittal sinus (SSS). Using a craniotome, a free bone flap is created.
- The SSS is separated under direct vision.
- The exposed SSS is covered with cottonoids and Surgicel.
- Tack-up sutures are placed before opening the dura.
- The dura is opened circumferentially around the tumour with the dural base on the SSS.
- The tumour is devascularized by isolating the blood supply and internally debulked by using the CUSA.
- Identify the arachnoid plane. The tumour is then dissected away from the surrounding brain. The area is covered with cottonoids.
- The tumour is then imploded and removed piecemeal.
- Careful attention must be paid to the arachnoid plane at the tumour–brain interface to make sure that no residual tumour is left behind (including dura and bone).
- Ensure adequate haemostasis.

Parasagittal/parafalcine meningioma

Key points and safety considerations

Image guidance.

Placement of craniotomy over the midline – safe burr holes (perforator over sinus vs. paramedian burr holes and drilling over the sinus).

Preservation of the draining veins.

Protection of anterior cerebral arteries deep to the tumour.

Total vs. near-total resection, if the sinus is invaded.

Potential pitfalls

Depending on imaging to establish sinus patency.

In cases of sinus occlusion, wide falcine resection compromising collateral venous channels within dural leaves.

Resection of infiltrated sinus and reconstruction. (Even in most expert hands significant precautions should be observed. Operation may not be considered at all in posterior half.)

Case 21

A 36-year-old woman presents with a chronic history of headaches. Her MRI scan demonstrates uniform enhancement of a space-occupying lesion in the lateral ventricle with mild hydrocephalus. She has been scheduled for surgery.

Intraventricular meningioma (posterior parieto-occipital transcortical approach)

- Preoperative angiogram with embolization may be required.
- General anaesthetic is employed.
- IV antibiotics are begun.
- Preoperative steroids and antibiotics are given and a urinary catheter is inserted.
- The patient is placed in a park bench position with head secured in a Mayfield 3-point pin fixation and elevated approximately 30°. When using the image guidance system, the tumour may be identified and marked on the patient's scalp.

- In selecting an entry point, the superior parietal eminence is used.
- A reverse U-shaped incision is used.
- A free bone flap is created.
- A Budde halo and microscope are used.
- The trajectory into the ipsilateral ventricle may be identified using an image guidance system and confirmed using a Dandy drainage cannula.
- Internal decompression of the tumour is performed using microsurgical techniques.
- A CUSA may help to minimize brain retraction.
- Occlusion of the choroidal artery branches should be achieved as early as possible.
- Careful attention is paid to the arachnoid plane at the tumour–brain interface to make sure that no residual tumour is left behind.
- Ensure adequate haemostasis.
- An EVD is inserted and remains *in situ* for the next 24 hours.

Case 22

A 48-year-old woman presents with thoracic pain and progressive lower limb weakness. She now walks with a stick. Her spinal MRI scan demonstrated an intradural extramedullary spinal tumour. She has been scheduled for surgery.

Debulking of an intradural spinal lesion (meningioma)

- Preoperative level marking may be performed by a radiologist.
- General anaesthetic is employed.
- Preoperative steroids and antibiotics are given and a urinary catheter is inserted.
- Intraoperative neurophysiology monitoring is recommended.
- The procedure is performed in a prone position on a Wilson frame, Montreal mattress or Jackson table. Pressure points are well protected.
- A linear midline incision is performed over the marked area.
- Both paraspinous muscles are stripped with monopolar diathermy.
- A laminectomy is performed ensuring the cranial and caudal end of the tumour is exposed. The tumour is usually visible underneath the arachnoid.
- The operating microscope is brought into the operative field.
- If the tumour is not visible, ultrasonography may be beneficial to evaluate the margins of the tumour. If inadequate exposure is seen, additional bone is removed to provide unobstructed surgical access.

- A linear durotomy is made and dural edges are hitched.
- The extent of the tumour is again examined.
- The tumour capsule is then coagulated with low voltage bipolar diathermy.
- The arachnoid is sharply divided and reflected to allow internal decompression of the tumour using either bipolar suction or CUSA.
- The plane between the tumour and spinal cord is then developed with progressive infolding of the tumour edges.
- Circumferential dissection in the arachnoid plane is continued until the tumour capsule is delivered in its entirety.
- The dural base is coagulated or excised.
- Adequate haemostasis must be ensured.

Resection of spinal meningioma

Key points and safety considerations

Correct localization of anatomical level.

Avoidance of manipulations of the spinal cord.

Possible benefits of intraoperative neurophysiological monitoring for extramedullary lesions.

Potential pitfalls

Consider division of the adjacent denticulate ligaments or sacrifice of a dorsal thoracic nerve root to gain access to an anterolaterally placed lesion rather than manipulating or retracting the spinal cord.

Prepare to discuss the case 'for or against' resection of the dural origin (e.g. true risk of recurrence vs dural repair and CSF leak).

Principles of operative surgery and surgical anatomy

A. Principles of intracranial aneurysm clipping

The emphasis is on safety and complication avoidance.

Position

Take into account the inclination of the skull base. Elevate the head. Avoid kinking of the jugular veins. Assess the degree of rotation and the location of the aneurysm to allow the temporal lobe to 'fall' away by gravity. For example, the position is more vertical for a laterally projecting posterior communicating artery (PCoA) aneurysm in order to approach the fundus and the position is more horizontal for a posteriorly projecting PCoA aneurysm in order to visualize the medial aspect of the aneurysm neck.

Craniotomy

Craniotomy should be large enough to allow access, angulations and different trajectories for the aneurysm clip. Usually, a more frontal exposure is required. Drill the sphenoid wing to minimize brain retraction. If you select a superciliary minicraniotomy (not recommended in an exam setting) then be prepared to address a premature aneurysm rupture and describe the use of special aneurysm clip applicators.

Brain relaxation

Lumbar drain

Beware of contraindication in the presence of associated intracranial haemorrhage (ICH).

EVD insertion

The EVD can be opened once the dura is opened to drain CSF from the basal cisterns. Drainage of CSF after incision and opening of the basal cisterns is the most common and effective way to achieve brain relaxation.

Ventricular puncture

Direct intraoperative ventricular puncture by aspiration of CSF should be considered, especially in the presence of ventriculomegaly and a swollen brain precluding access to the basal cisterns. The frontal horn is deep at the level of the inferior frontal gyrus. During a pterional craniotomy, the puncture point is 1–2 cm superior and 2–3 cm anterior to the anterior Sylvian point.

ICH evacuation

In the presence of a parenchymal ICH, partial evacuation of the haematoma, without eliminating the tamponade effect on the ruptured aneurysm, helps to achieve brain relaxation to access the basal cisterns and to achieve proximal control.

Basal cisterns

Opening the basal cisterns to drain CSF is important to help achieve brain relaxation.

Avoid brain retraction

Retraction injury should be avoided by adequate brain relaxation and CSF retrieval. Retractors, if used, act as brain 'holders' with only minimum pressure applied. Sharp dissection should be performed (e.g. splitting the Sylvian fissure). The direction of retraction and mobilization should be cautious in the following situations: (1) temporal lateral retraction in cases of laterally pointing PCoA aneurysms, (2) frontal superior retraction in cases of large inferiorly pointing ACoA aneurysms. In the former, the fundus may be adherent to the medial temporal lobe and in the latter the aneurysm may be adherent to the optic chiasm and lead to premature rupture.

Proximal control

This step must be mentioned in describing the overall procedure. In cases of MCA aneurysms, splitting of the Sylvian fissure widely exposes the M1 segment for proximal control. This also provides access to other territories (trans-Sylvian approach) and minimizes brain retraction. Special care should be given in preserving the perforators. In cases of temporary clip application, the perforators should be carefully dissected adjacent to the parent vessel to avoid their inclusion into the clip blades. For example, apply the temporary clip to the M1 distal to the origin of the lenticulostriate artery and in cases of applying the temporary clip to the A1 artery avoid inclusion of the recurrent artery of Heubner.

Neck dissection, clip application and preservation of distal branches

The identification of the aneurysm neck allows for clip placement and reduction in perforator injury. The aneurysm clip should be applied following full dissection of the aneurysm neck after adequate space is made for the insertion of the clip blades. An attempt to use the clip blades to dissect aneurysm may result in rupture or tearing of the aneurysm sac. The manufacturers indicate that the closing pressure is less at the tip of the blades. Ensure the clip blades are beyond the aneurysm neck. Multiple clip reconstruction may be required for wide-necked aneurysms. In selected cases, the use of appropriate fenestrated clips avoids kinking of distal branches and potential slippage. The clip should occlude the aneurysm, and allow patency of perforators and major branches. Intraoperative indocyanine green (ICG) fluorescence angiography is valuable in assessing the aneurysm exclusion and vessel patency.

Temporary clip application

During an intraoperative rupture, the application of temporary clips is necessary. They can also be used during the steps of neck dissection, particularly with friable aneurysms that are adherent to surrounding vessels. The temporary clip decreases the tension and slackens the sac to facilitate successful clip application. The closing pressure of temporary clips is less than for the definitive clip. Nevertheless, avoid application of the clip on a parent vessel with an atheromatous segment because this may lead to a plaque 'break' and formation of a thromboembolism. Preserve the perforators. When clipping an M1 aneurysm avoid compromising the lumen of the MCA branches, including the lenticulostriate arteries. Likewise, when clipping an A1 aneurysm, preserve the recurrent artery of Heubner. In cases of prolonged temporary clip application, ensure neuroprotection: head elevation, maintenance perfusion blood pressure and adequate oxygenation and sedation (e.g. mannitol and propofol). In cases of SAH, the tolerability is variable and depends on the vulnerability of neural tissue and the vessel itself (less tolerated for the basilar artery aneurysm). The duration of temporary clip application may be guided by monitoring techniques, such as SSEPs.

Avoid intraoperative aneurysm rupture

Measures to avoid rupture include anaesthetic techniques, limited brain retraction, proximal control, application of temporary clips and proper dissection of the aneurysm neck. Ensure the patient remains haemodynamically stable. Maintain a stable blood pressure with appropriate anaesthesia and adequate analgesia. The anatomy of the aneurysm should be appreciated. For example, aggressive temporal retraction may result in premature rupture of a laterally projecting PCoA aneurysm with its fundus adherent to the temporal lobe. In addition, superior retraction on the frontal lobe may tear an inferiorly projecting ACoA aneurysm with fundus adherent to the optic chiasm or optic nerve. Complete the neck dissection prior to clip application. Perform sharp dissection of arachnoid adhesions to prevent the clip blades from tearing the fundus. Apply a temporary clip if the aneurysm sac appears tense. Intraoperative rupture can occur during any stage of the operation. This is most challenging if it occurs before access to the parent vessel. This will necessitate aggressive anaesthetic measures to combat brain swelling in order to obtain control. Moreover, neuroprotection is also required with prolonged temporary clip application. Full identification and dissection of the aneurysm neck is required – a hasty clip application may lead to premature rupture.

B. Principles of intrinsic glioma resection

The emphasis is on understanding the neuro anatomy, recent technical advances and controversies.

Image-guidance systems

Image-guidance systems are used routinely in neurosurgery. To establish a histological diagnosis, image-guided biopsies are performed. Image guidance helps the surgeon to select the shortest route from the cortical surface and avoid traversing the ventricular cavities and vascular areas (e.g. Sylvian fissure and pineal region). In cases of glioma resection, image guidance helps to confirm the underlying anatomy, delineate tumour margins and demonstrate white matter tracts (with the use of tractography).

Awake craniotomy

Different anaesthetic techniques including local anaesthesia and sedation or 'asleep – awake – asleep' techniques using general anaesthesia with intraoperative wake-up can be used. Electrophysiological mapping includes frequency of stimulation, cortical and white matter tract stimulation, and speech and motor assessments. Awake craniotomy is safe and well tolerated. Be aware of the safety topics: airway protection, avoidance and management of intraoperative seizures, vomiting and pain control. Be prepared to debate the merits of this approach compared to other options (intraoperative MRI).

Intraoperative monitoring

Resection of intrinsic lesions is a favourite exam question and assesses your neuroanatomical knowledge. Describe the lesion in relation to the sulcus and gyrus. The choice of trajectory is selected to indicate your anatomical knowledge, including eloquent areas and white matter tracts. Intraoperative monitoring is a surgical adjunct to aid in your resection. Demonstrate knowledge of the neurophysiological parameters, frequency of stimulation, design of the bipolar stimulators and types of recordings. For example, motor responses are recorded by clinical assessment or neurophysiological monitoring. Speech responses (including higher mental function) require experienced neurologists, neuropsychologists, or speech and language therapists. You should be aware of the variation in amplitude and frequency of stimulation in assessing the white matter tracts. You should express your knowledge of the anatomy, orientation and projection of the white matter tracts.

Ultrasound

Ultrasound uses high-frequency sound waves to create an image. The advantages include availability and real-time imaging. Disadvantages include surgeon dependence and limited resolution.

5-Aminolevulinic acid (5-ALA)

5-ALA is a porphyrin-based compound that does not cross an intact blood–brain barrier and is selectively taken up into malignant glial cells. The 'dye' is activated with light at the near-blue spectrum and fluoresces by emitting wavelengths near the red spectrum. It is detected by filters mounted on the operative microscope.

Cavitron ultrasonic surgical aspirator (CUSA)

The ultrasonic waves induces shock waves, bubbling and cavitation to the intracellular water content coupled with expansion, evaporation and disruption of cells. CUSA can be selected for firm lesions to help reduce intraoperative bleeding and perioperative morbidity. CUSA has a limited value in debulking extremely calcified or dense fibrous lesions. The heat generated may also be detrimental to the adjacent neural structures.

Gliadel wafers

You may be asked to describe their chemical composition (polifeprosan 20 with carmustine implant), relative contraindications (open ventricles), potential side effects (e.g. seizures, brain oedema, delayed wound healing and intracranial infections) and indications in newly diagnosed and recurrent high-grade malignant gliomas. Be aware of the surgical techniques of placement of the wafers and importance of dural closure.

C. Principles of microsurgical resection of arteriovenous malformations

Operative planning

Review the imaging (MRI scan and angiogram) to assess the nidal anatomy, obtain critical information regarding the major feeding vessels and draining veins, identify arteries *en passage* and establish if a cortical arteriovenous malformation (AVM) is based on the ventricle.

Compartments

Arterial

The angiogram assesses the filling of the nidus by different vascular territories demonstrated by different injections. Do not rely on one injection. On reviewing the carotid injection, it is possible to underestimate the extent of the AVM if it is supplied by distal MCA or anterior cerebral artery (ACA) branches.

Venous

Multiple draining veins are common. However, in a few cases, compartmentalization of the nidus may occur with each segment predominantly draining into a different draining vein. Preoperatively, the appreciation of this arrangement allows for the surgeon to plan to expose all the draining veins and allow for complete resection.

Nidus location

The location of the nidus determines the 'eloquence' of the AVM and predicts the patient's potential post-operative neurological deficits. An MRI scan demonstrates its relationship to the cortical regions and plans the trajectory (e.g. transsulcal approach for subcortical lesions) The AVM's relationship to white matter tracts can been seen by tractography and its relationship to functional neural tissue can been by fMRI imaging. One limitation of fMRI imaging is that the signal adjacent to the abnormal blood flow through the nidus may be difficult to determine.

Feeders

Knowledge of angiographic anatomy enables the surgeon to determine the location of the main feeders (e.g. the two terminal branches of the PCA are located in the calcarine and occipito-parietal sulci).

Draining veins

Knowing the location of the surface draining veins is the key to intraoperative localization of the nidus. The location of the deep venous drainage would identify the deep extent of the nidus.

Craniotomy

Plan the craniotomy. A large flap is recommended in the following instances:

- AVM nidus cannot be retracted as much as the surgeon would often like
- The nidus cannot be gutted from within.
- The surface veins may further restrict one's access to the base of the malformation.
- Adequate identification of surface clues is needed.
- The draining vein on the surface needs to be traced retrogradely to locate the subcortical nidus.

Skeletonization of vessels

The initial dissection aims to access the arterial feeders, identify the draining veins and access the nidus. The covering arachnoidal membrane has to be meticulously incised to expose the adequate segments of the vessels circumferentially.

Identification of draining veins

The arterialized draining veins are initially preserved because premature occlusion of these veins may result in significant and troublesome bleeding secondary to an increase in the intranidal pressure. The veins act as a 'gauge'. Their collapse and colour change (returning to venous dark blue) indicates adequate obliteration of the nidus, and only then can the AVM be disconnected and subsequently removed.

Resection of nidus

Cautery and interruption of feeding vessels is required. Use bipolar coagulation perpendicular to the vessels. Ensure you are constantly moving around the AVM to ensure your dissection is performed evenly (avoid deep holes). Apply Surgicel and cottonoids to help establish the brain–AVM interface. Once the dissected cavity is a few centimetres deep, place a temporary clip on the major feeder to help establish that it is terminating in one nidus. This will also help decrease the tension within the AVM. In addition, cortical AVMs are based on the ventricle. Secure the ventricle and address the choroidal and ependymal feeders. Once the test occlusion is complete, a permanent aneurysmal clip is placed on the main draining vein.

En-passage feeders

These feeders should be respected, perhaps leaving a temporary clip and only dividing the feeders that terminate in the nidus.

Finale

Ensure adequate haemostasis throughout the surgery. Small feeders that are not adequately coagulated may retract and result in parenchymal intracerebral haematoma. Test the resection bed for breakthrough bleeding. Breakthrough bleeding can be evidence of retained AVM or disrupted autoregulation in the surrounding tissue. Persistent bleeding from the AVM bed usually indicates a residual nidus. In such cases, the nidus should be explored and resected accordingly.

D. Principles of trauma craniotomy

Craniotomy

For small and moderate acute subdural and extradural haematomas, the craniotomy should be tailored to encompass the margins of the haematoma. In cases of fracture haematomas, the craniotomy should circumscribe areas of a comminuted skull fracture to allow the bone fragments to be fixed together with mini-plates.

For large subdural and extradural haematomas associated with diffuse head injuries, a large frontotemporoparietal craniotomy allows for adequate decompression of the haematoma, haemostasis and brain swelling.

Acute extradural haematoma

This surgical procedure is expected to be described in detailed during the examination. Be aware of the challenging questions related to the techniques for bleeding (including intraoperative coagulopathy), brain swelling, dural laceration and torn sinuses.

Acute subdural haematoma

Acute subdural haematomas are commonly associated with severe head injuries. The traumatic forces disrupt the underlying brain tissue and the bridging veins. The haematoma can be associated with underlying brain contusions (including a 'burst' temporal lobe). In these cases, a decompressive craniectomy is required to address the haematoma, brain swelling and increased intracranial pressure.

Contusions

Contusions can be located deep and superficial to the brain's surface. Deep-seated contusions that extend to the cortical surface may incorporate viable and functional neural tissue. Cortical location and time from injury have implications in surgical planning. In cases of multiple contusions and persistent increased intracranial pressure, a decompressive craniectomy may be considered.

Intraoperative swelling

Intraoperative swelling can occur throughout surgery: at the time of dural opening, clot evacuation or closure. In these cases recommend the following:

- Elevate the patient's head.
- Optimize the anaesthetic parameters (ensure adequate oxygenation, ventilation and sedation; treat with mannitol and brief moderate hyperventilation).
- Effect rapid evacuation of the haematoma.
- Coagulate bleeding vessels.
- Assess for a reversible cause – residual haematoma. If ultrasound is available, this may identify a deep intracerebral ICH or, rarely, an interhemispheric subdural haematoma.
- Leave the dura open (with or without a dural substitute).
- Check to see if insertion of an ICP bolt and immediate post-operative CT scan is recommended.

E. Principles of specialized disorders

Movement disorders

- Ensure knowledge of the disorder: the clinical features, pathophysiology, neurotransmitters and management.
- Know the principles of stereotaxy and the different types of stereotactic frames.
- Plan target and trajectory: stimulation in awake patients, stereotaxic atlases, Tesla (3T) MRI imaging including tractography and microelectrode recordings.
- Know the surgical steps: create burr hole, open dura and pia maters, advance electrode (check impedance), ± obtain electrode recordings and stimulation, and implant deep brain stimulation (DBS).

Epilepsy

- Operative planning includes the following:
  - Confirmation of the diagnosis (e.g. exclude pseudoseizures).
  - Establishing indications for surgery (frequency, quality of life, medical intractable seizures).
  - Localize the focus (non-invasive vs. invasive-grid and depth electrodes).

- List types of surgery (palliative, resections and stimulation).
- Review investigations: imaging (MRI, fMRI, PET, ictal and interictal SPECT), Wada testing, neuropsychological testing and electroencephalographic (EEG) findings.

■ Demonstrate knowledge regarding neuro-anatomical principles of temporal lobectomy, extratemporal resections, subpial transections, vagal nerve stimulator (VNS) insertion, anatomy and approaches to choroid plexus, choroid fissure, hippocampus and amygdala. Discuss surgery outcome scales.

Engel epilepsy surgery outcome scale

- Class I: Free of disabling seizures.
- Class II: Rare disabling seizures ('almost seizure-free').
- Class III: Worthwhile improvement.
- Class IV: No worthwhile improvement.

Spasticity

■ Demonstrate knowledge regarding aetiology, pathophysiology, grading systems (see Table 4.2) and treatments of spasticity.

Table 4.2 Ashworth grading system for spasticity

Grade	Description
0	No increase in muscle tone.
1	Slight increase in muscle tone, manifested by a catch and release or by minimal resistance at the end of the range of motion when the affected part(s) is moved in flexion or extension.
1+	Slight increase in muscle tone, manifested by a catch, followed by minimal resistance throughout the remainder (less than half) of the ROM.
2	More marked increase in muscle tone through most of the ROM, but affected part(s) easily moved.
3	Considerable increase in muscle tone, passive movement difficult.
4	Affected part(s) rigid in flexion or extension.

- Medical options include diazepam, baclofen, dantrolene, and progabide.
- Surgical options include botulinum injections, intrathecal baclofen, electrical stimulation via epidural electrodes, selective dorsal rhizotomy, intramuscular phenol neurolyis, myelotomies, stereotactic thalamotomy or dentatomy.

Carotid artery stenosis

■ Demonstrate awareness of evidence-based trials regarding the indications for carotid endarterectomy: Asymptomatic Carotid Surgery Trial (ACST), Asymptomatic Carotid Atherosclerosis Study (ACAS), Veterans Affairs Cooperative Study (VACS), European Carotid Surgery Trial (ECST) and North American Symptomatic Carotid Endarterectomy Trial (NACET) (for full details, see Chapter 7: Landmark Publications).

■ State anatomical landmarks and important structures encountered during the procedure, including platysma, fascial planes, carotid sheath, carotid arteries (common, external and internal), carotid sinus, recurrent laryngeal nerve, vagus nerve, marginal mandibular branch of facial nerve, ansa cervicalis and hypoglossal nerve.

■ Discuss intraoperative monitoring: transcranial Doppler (TCD) and EEG.

■ Note controversies: selective or routine intraoperative intraluminal shunting, patient selection and carotid artery stenting.

CSF leakage

■ State aetiology of CSF leakage including cranial and spinal pathology (traumatic, spontaneous, congenital, iatrogenic, medication [dopamine agonists]).

■ Discuss preoperative imaging: CT and MRI.

■ List principles of CSF surgical repair.
- Cranial approaches: craniotomy and endoscopic intranasal approach and the use of intraoperative dyes (fluorescein) during the repair.
- Spinal approaches: open repair and shunting.

■ Do not forget to use prophylactic Pneumovax, when appropriate.

Peripheral neuropathies

- Definitions.
  Peripheral neuropathy: diffuse lesions of peripheral nerves producing weakness, sensory disturbance and/or reflex changes.
  Mononeuropathy: a disorder of a single nerve, often attributed to trauma or entrapment.
  Mononeuropathy multiplex: involvement of two or more nerves, usually due to a systemic abnormality.
- Aetiology of peripheral neuropathies. Use the mnemonic: **ABCDEFGHI**

A	Alcoholism
	Amyloid
	AIDS
	Acute intermittent porphyria
B	B12 deficiency
C	Chronic inflammatory demyelinating polyneuropathy
	Connective tissue disorders (polyarteritis nodosa, rheumatoid arthritis, systematic lupus erythematosus)

D	Diabetes
	Drugs (vincristine, dexamethasone, statins, metronidazole, phenytoin, amitriptyline)
	Diphtheria
E	Endocrine
	Entrapment
	Environmental toxins (organophosphate)
F	Thyroid disorders (hypothyroidism – carpal tunnel syndrome, hyperthyroidism – polyneuropathy)
G	Guillain–Barré syndrome
H	Hereditary (Charot-Marie-Tooth disease)
I	Infection (Leprosy – Hansen's disease)

- The clinical features of the following neuropathies are important: brachial plexus injuries, median nerve entrapment, ulnar nerve entrapment and radial nerve entrapment.
- Classification of peripheral nerve injuries: Seddon system (1943) and Sunderland system (1951) (see Table 4.3).

Table 4.3 Peripheral nerve injuries: Seddon and Sunderland classifications of peripheral nerve injury

Sunderland	Seddon	Description of injury	Recovery period
I	Neurapraxia	Conduction block, nerve is in-continuity, Wallerian degeneration does not take place	≤ 3 months
II	Axonotmesis	Axon not continuous, nerve itself remains intact, axonal sprouting, Wallerian degeneration	1 inch [25.4 mm] per month
III		During healing, excessive scarring of the endoneurium occurs that hinders axon regeneration	< 1 inch per month where it is slowed by the scar tissue; determined by degree of scarring and involved fascicles
IV		Nerve is still in-continuity, scar build-up blocks nerve regeneration	Surgical intervention required to reestablish nerve transduction by removing scar tissue and reconnecting nerve segments
V	Neurotmesis	Rupture of the nerve, it is no longer a continuous fibre	Recovery requires surgical intervention

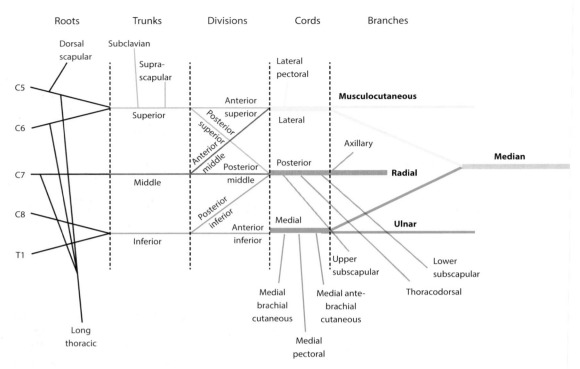

Figure 4.5 Schematic diagram of the nerves of the brachial plexus

- *Nerve growth factor (NGF)* is a secreted protein that promotes differentiation, growth, maintenance, and survival of certain target neurons. They have an important role in signalling, neuroprotection and repair.

The emphasis of this section of the examination is your neuroanatomical knowledge, safety and complication avoidance.

The viva: investigation of the neurosurgical patient including neuroradiology and neuropathology

Introduction

This may be the most straightforward section of the examination and it is easy to score good marks.

In a viva setting, remember this is a neurosurgical rather than a radiology examination. Imagine that you are communicating the results of the radiological images with a neurosurgeon over the telephone in order to plan the operation. Describe the radiological images to establish the differential diagnosis, the anatomical location of the lesion (deep vs. superficial), ease of surgery, possible complications, and timing of surgery based on mass effect and herniation.

When describing an image, it is important to mention the type of investigation, verifying the patient's demographic details (name and date of birth) and date the investigation took place. For computed tomography (CT) and magnetic resonance imaging (MRI) scans, report if the lesion is intra- or extra-axial. Is there evidence of contrast enhancement? This will narrow the list of differential diagnoses. Be precise about the anatomical

location of the lesion. It is best to avoid general terms, such as 'brainstem'; be specific: midbrain tectum, pons or medulla oblongata. Similarly, locate the lesion by its lobe, gyrus and sulcus. In addition, for deep-seated lesions mention the adjacent white matter tracts. This will allow your management to be safe and clear (surgical vs. non-surgical management; biopsy vs. subtotal vs. total resections; and potential complications of treatment). Include descriptions of mass effect, perilesional oedema and hydrocephalus.

MRI scan interpretation – sample answer

This axial MRI scan T1-weighted image without contrast demonstrates large solitary well-defined heterogeneous/variable intensity mass in the right/left frontal lobe adjacent to____. There is also associated surrounding oedema and mass effect as evidenced by the sulci effacement and compression of the ____ ventricle. These features are suggestive of ____although other differentials include____. (See Table 5.1 for the differential diagnosis of intracranial lesions.)

Table 5.1   Differential diagnosis of intracranial lesions based on anatomical location, +/- enhancement and +/- surrounding oedema

Location		Enhancement	Lesion	Oedema
Supra-tentorial	Extra-axial	+	Meningioma	±
		+	Metastasis	+
		-	Arachnoid cyst	-
		-	Epidermoid cyst	-
	Intra-axial	+	High grade glioma	+
		+	Pilocytic astrocytoma	-
		+	Metastasis	++
		+	Cerebral lymphoma	+
		-	Low-grade glioma	-
	Sella/suprasellar	+	Pituitary adenoma	-
		+	Craniopharyngioma	±
		-	Rathke's cleft cyst	-
		±	Optic nerve glioma	±
	Intra-ventricular	+	Colloid cyst	
		+	Glioma/central neurocytoma	N/A
		+	Meningioma	N/A
		+	Choroid plexus papilloma	N/A
		+	Ependymoma	N/A
		-	Subependymoma	N/A
Infra-tentorial	Extra-axial	+	Meningioma	±
		+	Schwannoma	-
		-	Epidermoid cyst	-
	Intra-axial	+	Metastasis	++
		+	Medulloblastoma	+
		+	Pilocytic astrocytoma	-
		+	Haemangioblastoma	-
		+	Brainstem glioma	±
	Intra-ventricular	+	Ependymoma	N/A
		+	Choroid plexus papilloma	N/A

Targeted differential diagnosis

Having studied tables and lists of differential diagnoses from textbooks, you may be surprised that when shown a radiological image the vast majority of the list of differential diagnoses does not apply. Starting your answer with 'There are many possibilities to explain this image...' and then finding out that there are only two potential diagnoses may lead to a difficult situation. For example, the list of differential diagnoses of a vascular blush on a cerebral angiogram includes vascular malformations, dural arteriovenous fistula (DAVF), renal cell metastases, haemangiopericytoma or haemangioblastoma. However, if the angiogram depicts a large arteriovenous malformation (AVM) in the parietal lobe, with feeding arteries leading to a tangled nidus that shunts blood directly into a large draining vein, there is only one diagnosis. Therefore, it is best to provide a short list of possible differential diagnoses and explain your reasoning.

Management justification

This is not a separate exam component, but rather it is one of the purposes, if not the main purpose, of oral and clinical examination. Management is an important feature in the investigation viva. Therefore, after formulating a diagnosis, treatment options should be discussed. It is best to list all the treatment modalities (conservative, medical, radiological and surgical) and then place the emphasis on the most important treatments. In the viva, presenting a balanced view may be a challenge. Do not appear hesitant or flippant. Remember it is best to recommend the safe and standard treatment options.

Principles of radiology

In this section you may also be asked about principles of radiology:

- CT scan.
- MRI scan.
- Single-photon emission computed tomography (SPECT) scan.
- Positron emission tomography (PET) scan.

- **CT scan** – utilizes X-ray beam, which traverses the patient's head, diametrically opposed detector that measures the extent of resorption.
- **MRI scan** – superimposed electromagnetic pulse (radio waves) at specific frequency displaces the hydrogen atom.
  - **T1** – spin lattice relaxation. The time taken for protons to realign themselves with magnetic field.
  - **T2** – spin to spin relaxation. The time taken for protons to return to their out of phase state.
  - **Diffusion weighted** – thermally driven translational movement of water.
  - **Functional** – T2 relaxation time of perfused brain – oxy Hb. A mismatch of O_2 supply and utilization in the activated area causes signal change due to blood-oxygenation-level-dependent (BOLD).
  - **Perfusion** – bolus tracking after rapid contrast injection.
- **SPECT scan.**
  - Uses compounds labelled with gamma emitting tracers.
- **PET scan.**
  - Utilizes positron-emitting isotope bound compound.
  - Need a cyclotron for production.
  - To assess relationship of cerebral blood flow (CBF) and O_2 demand.

Case scenarios

Case 1

A 15-year-old girl presents with acute worsening headaches with a background history of progressive lower limb weakness.

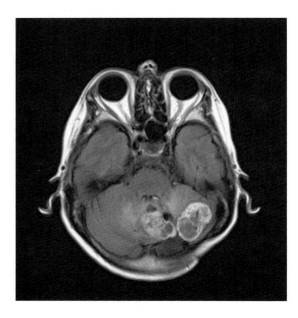

Please describe the anomaly shown.

This axial T1WI MRI scan demonstrates left cerebellar cystic lesions with enhancing mural nodule and compression of the 4th ventricle. There is evidence of surrounding oedema.

Tips

You may also mention this:

'If available, I would also like to review the complete unenhanced images to ensure the patient doesn't have hydrocephalus'.

Remember this patient has headaches and progressive lower limb weakness. Why? The next question could be the following.

What could have been the cause for her presentation?

Headache. Hydrocephalus, other supratentorial haemangioblastoma.

Paraparesis. Cerebellar lesion, motor cortex lesions, spinal cord lesions.

What is your provisional and differential diagnosis?

- Cerebellar haemangioblastoma.
- Pilocystic astrocytoma.

What are the relevant clinical examinations and investigations that would follow the urgent treatment of this patient?

The relevant clinical examination would include the following:

- Fundoscopy and slit lamp examination by the ophthalmologist for retinal angiomas.
- Blood pressure measurement for phaeochromocytoma.
- Full blood count for polycythaemia.
- MRI scan of the whole neuroaxis for concurrent haemangioblastoma in the brain and spinal cord and endolymphatic cyst.
- CT scan thorax/abdomen/pelvis for solid organ tumours and cyst.

If the patient was diagnosed to be positive for von Hippel–Lindau (VHL) disease, who else should be screened?

I would screen all first-degree relatives.

The normal age for screening is as follows:

- 5 years: ophthalmology review annually.
- 10 years: urine for vanillylmendelic acid (VMA) and homovanillic acid (HCA) annually.
- 15 years: abdominal ultrasound/MRI abdomen annually.
- 19 years: CNS MRI scanning and then annually.

An undiagnosed adult will be screened for all of these.

I would arrange genetic counselling and educate the patient on VHL. If she plans to become pregnant, I would engage an obstetrician and highlight the relevance of contraception, pre-implantation genetic counselling and abortion.

On her spinal MRI scan, multiple avidly enhancing lesions were seen. How would you manage these lesions?

I would be guided by clinical and radiological features. If the lesions were causing progressive paraparesis, then I would discuss the options with the patient about resection of the relevant lesions;

otherwise I would monitor them at a regular interval depending on the clinical picture.

If the brain lesion was an incidental finding, how would you approach the situation?

I would discuss the options with patient and family and screen her for VHL. Given an option, I advise surgical resection because there is evidence of fourth ventricular compression and possible hydrocephalus. I would also be guided by complete clinical examination, and I would look for early signs of cerebellar and brainstem compression.

Case 2

A 36-year-old woman, who is 24 weeks pregnant, presents with persistent headaches, vomiting and bilateral papilloedema. She is alert and orientated.

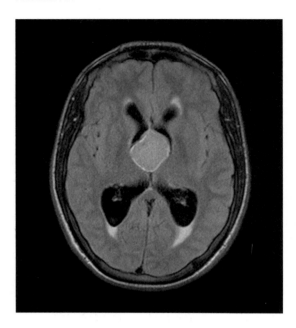

What is the diagnosis?

This is an axial MRI of the head that shows a hyperdense lesion at the level of the foramen of Monro causing biventricular hydrocephalus. This is most likely due to a colloid cyst.

What would your management options be?

The key clinical problems are the following:

1. The patient is facing a life-threatening condition secondary to hydrocephalus.
2. She is pregnant with a viable fetus. There is a need for an urgent multidisciplinary discussion with the obstetrician (fetal-maternal specialist), neonatologist, obstetric anaesthetist and intensivist. If the patient's condition deteriorates, there is an option of delivering the baby, although prematurely through a caesarean section.

The patient was scheduled for an endoscopic resection of the cyst. When the introducer was removed, the camera did not reveal any recognizable structures and there were no visible vessels. What do you think happened?

The camera was probably within the cavum septum pellucidum and needs to be readjusted.

Case 3

A 25-year-old man is involved in a road traffic accident and brought into the emergency department comatose.

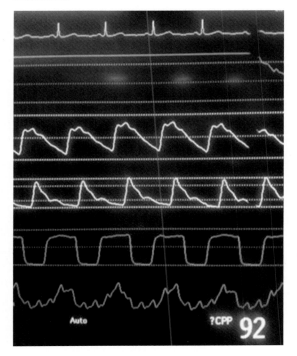

Please identify the intracranial pressure (ICP) waveforms.

The third wave from the top.

What is the abnormality here? Please describe what each peak may represent.

The P2 is greater than P1: this would represent a non-compliant brain in a high ICP setting (intracranial hypertension).

P1: percussion wave - represents arterial pulsation.

P2: tidal wave - represents intracranial compliance.

P3: dicrotic wave - represents aortic valve closure.

In healthy patients, the height of P1>P2>P3.

What are the possible methods of ICP measurements?

Clinical monitoring is very important and reliable.

- The most common method in a neurosurgical setting is with an ICP monitor. This can be achieved by direct methods of measurement using an intraventricular device, e.g. using an external ventricular drain (EVD) and attaching it to a transducer (the gold standard, which has therapeutic advantages).

- Other methods include the use of microtransducer devices and placing them in the following areas:
  - Parenchyma (most common).
  - Subarachnoid.
  - Subdural.
  - Epidural and lumbar spine.
- The devices used are broadly divided into the following:
  - Piezoelectric strain gauge devices (Codman).
  - Fibreoptic (Camino).
  - Pneumatic sensors (Spiegelberg).

The pneumatic device does not need zeroing and calibrates itself every hour. There is a risk of zero drifting that may affect the accuracy of the device.

- Indirect methods of measurement can be used as well.
  - Transcranial Doppler (TCD).
  - Tympanic membrane displacement.
  - Optic neural sheath diameter.
  - Fundoscopy (Frisen scale), although this is less accurate and not widely used in clinical practice.

The patient is in the intensive care unit (ICU) and ventilated with deep sedation. What method of cerebral oxygenation determination could be used in this situation?

Jugular bulb oximetry uses fibre-optic technology to detect the spectrum of light absorption of oxyhaemoglobin. Alternatively, a jugular puncture can be performed or a venous catheter could be passed to place the tip on the jugular bulb. This could be performed on the side of brain injury where there is dominant venous drainage (debatable). Cerebral oximetry (near-infrared spectroscopy) can be beneficial.

What methods of measurement of cerebral blood flow (CBF) are you aware of?

$$CBF = \frac{\text{cerebral perfusion pressure (CPP)}}{\text{cerebrovascular resistance (CVR)}}$$

- Clinical examination and consciousness level (Glasgow coma scale [GCS]).
- TCD.
- Katy and Schmidt's method based on the Fick principle using an Xe-133 CT scan.
- PET scan to measure a specific body process or function. A radiolabelled substance is

injected into the body. Positrons are released and detected by a camera that builds a three-dimensional (3D) image.

■ SPECT scan – radioactive substance that measures CBF, releases gamma rays that are detected by a gamma camera, which builds a 3D image.

■ CT perfusion.

■ MR perfusion.

What other direct method of measurement could be used to measure cerebral metabolism in this patient?

Microdialysis utilizes Ringer's lactate at the rate of 0.3 microlitres/minute through a semipermeable membrane. The dialysate is extracted and assessed for the following products: lactate, lactate/pyruvate ratio, glycerol, glucose and glutamate.

Case 4

A 50-year-old woman with known renal failure presents with a sudden severe headache.

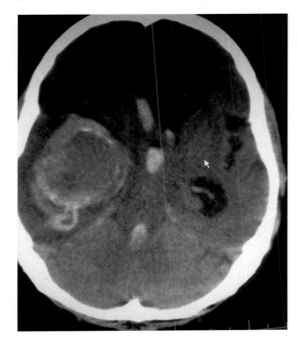

Please describe the scan. What is the diagnosis and the differential diagnosis?

Plain CT head scan demonstrates a large heterogeneous right-sided globular shaped mass with evidence of peripheral calcification. There is some fresh haemorrhage that has extended into the ventricular system. The mass effect and bleed seem to have occluded the right foramen of Monro causing contralateral dilated ventricles. There is an abnormal projection from the mass posteriorly; a giant aneurysm should be considered as a primary diagnosis. The differential diagnoses are a large temporal abscess or tumour (which can be primary or secondary).

What other types of imaging may help to diagnose the condition?

CT angiogram/digital subtraction angiogram.

The lesion was treated surgically with a high-flow bypass and clipping. How would the patient be followed up as outpatient?

She can be followed up with serial scans. The available options are computer to screen (CTS) imaging, magnetic resonance angiography (MRA) and digital subtraction angiography (DSA). This would depend on the local hospital's policy because all are acceptable methods with their own merits and risks. Because the patient had surgical treatment based on the ISAT trial, there is a lower incidence of recurrence as compared to coiling. I would prefer to perform an MRA using the time of flight sequence, which eliminates the risk of contrast nephropathy because the patient has renal failure.

The patient became more drowsy on day 5 after surgery. What are the relevant investigations necessary in this situation?

Obtain complete history, perform the clinical examination and assess the vital signs. This would include arterial blood gases (ABGs), blood pressure (BP), temperature and fluid balance.

The following causes with their appropriate investigations should be considered:

- Hyponatraemia secondary to syndrome of inappropriate antidiuretic hormone secretion (SIADH) or cerebral salt wasting (CSW) – serum sodium.
- Pneumonia or pulmonary emboli secondary to inadequate oxygenation and lung complications – ABG and electrocardiography (ECG).
- Urinary tract infection (UTI) – urine microscopy.
- Hydrocephalus – urgent CT brain scan.
- Re-haemorrhage secondary to hyperperfusion breakthrough or failed vascular anastomosis – urgent CT brain.
- Delayed cerebral ischaemia and infarction from inadequate bypass – SPECT scan, CT/MRI perfusion, MRI with diffusion-weighted imaging (DWI).
- Cerebral vasospasm – TCD.
- Seizure (non-convulsive/convulsive) – electroencephalography (EEG) and SPECT scan for interictal images.

How is TCD useful in aneurysmal rupture?

TCD uses the Doppler principle and can measure the following: heart rate (HR), peak volume, pulsatility index, end-diastolic velocity and Lindegaard ratio.

Lindegaard ratio = mean velocity in the middle cerebral artery (MCA) divided by mean velocity in ipsilateral extracranial internal carotid artery.

- High velocities in the MCA (>120 cm/s) may be due to hyperaemia or vasospasm.

- The Lindegaard ratio helps distinguish these conditions:
  - <3: hyperaemia.
  - >3: vasospasm (3–6: mild; >6: severe).

Three main windows are used: the temporal, suboccipital and orbital.

In approximately 10% of patients a temporal window produces inadequate insonation (ultrasound cannot penetrate the temporal bone).

The artery is identified by the direction of flow and depth.

- MCA: 6 cm and flow toward probe at 55 cm/s.
- ACA: 5 cm flow away from probe at 50 cm/s.
- PCA: 5 cm and flow toward the probe with a velocity of 40 cm/s.

The patient's identical twin sister approached you and is concerned about having a similar lesion herself and is keen to be investigated. How would you advise her?

If the patient is very anxious, a scan could be performed. There is a slight increase in aneurysm incidence among identical twins. However, there are merits and disadvantages. A screening tool, such as a CTA, may be done. The scan is not 100% sensitive in identifying all aneurysms and therefore a small proportion could be missed that could potentially rupture in the future. Because the natural history of aneurysm is still poorly understood, a negative scan does not mean that an aneurysm will not develop in the future. An aneurysm that is found may not rupture. However, a positive finding may put the clinician and patient in a dilemma because treatment itself is not risk-free. The level of anxiety may increase and this may affect the patient's lifestyle, occupation, driving, travel, insurance, and so forth. With a positive result, the patient may undergo serial imaging, which carries a risk of radiation. There is no clear consensus on how an aneurysm may be managed although there are guidelines. The treatment options are surgery or endovascular embolization. Some patients may be monitored.

Case 5

A 46-year-old teacher was admitted to the neurosurgical ward with a recent onset of cognitive decline and headache. An MRI brain scan demonstrates a contrast-enhancing solitary lesion adjacent to the occipital horn of the left ventricle. She underwent a frameless-based biopsy of the underlying lesion.

Describe the histology slide.

This shows an area of hypercellularity with marked hyperchromatism and pleomorphism. There is also prominent vascularity and an area of palisading necrosis.

What is the diagnosis?

Glioblastoma multiforme.

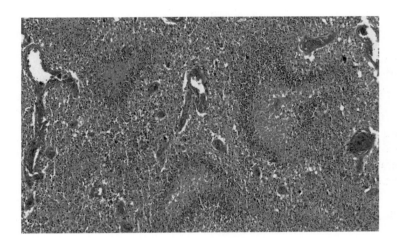

Case 6

A 26-year-old newsreader was assaulted and presents with a GCS of 13/15 (E3V4M6).

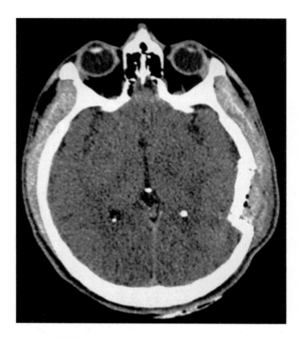

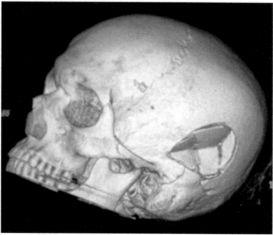

Where is the abnormality? What is the immediate management?

The patient has a depressed skull fracture on the left temporo-parietal region. There is a small contusion underlying the fracture. I would ensure that the patient had a complete primary and secondary survey and is started on anticonvulsants.

There was no wound. How would you manage this patient?

I would be guided by the patient's neurological status. Because there is no open wound, this is not a neurosurgical emergency. This may be potentially managed conservatively. I would engage the patient in this decision.

What neurological deficits could be present?

Right-sided hemiparesis and dysphasia.

The patient was managed in the ICU and was localizing to pain; however, he had regular episodes of unexplained neurological deterioration. How would you investigate this?

I would consider nonconvulsive seizures. I would check the serum glucose and perform an EEG.

There was a new onset of progressive dysphasia. A repeat CT scan demonstrated localized oedema. His family was inquiring if surgery could be helpful in reversing this and controlling seizures.

Surgery could be undertaken for progressive neurological deficit, and this may reverse. However, there is no convincing evidence about improving seizure control.

He was discharged home and presented 6 weeks later with an episode of generalized seizure. What are the possible causes for this event?

The patient may be developing late-onset posttraumatic seizures (PTS) secondary to his head injury. Other possibilities are intracranial abscess, subdural empyema and venous sinus thrombosis.

Case 7

A 13-year-old girl presents with worsening gait and frequent falls at school.

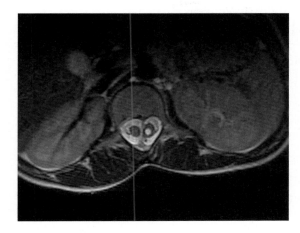

What is the abnormality?

A split cord abnormality with a median septum.

What is the diagnosis?

Split cord malformation (SCM).

Why could the patient be experiencing neurological deterioration?

During growth spurts, patients may deteriorate as a result of pressure on the spinal cord.

What preoperative investigations and imaging are necessary?

- Complete MRI imaging of neuraxis.
- CT myelography.
- MRI of abdomen at the level of the lesion (SCM may be associated with neurenteric cyst).
- Urodynamic testing.

The patient was found to have a low-lying conus medullaris. Why is this important from a surgical point of view?

There may be an associated tethered cord. This is important because the orthopaedic team may be considering scoliosis correction and it would require neurosurgical involvement.

There are two different situations that need to be addressed: a tethered cord and the diastometomyelia.

Which should be treated first and why?

It is safer to treat the SCM first. If detethering the cord is done instead, there is a risk of the cord shearing when it moves cranially through a rigid bony septum.

If this were an isolated incidental finding, would it need treatment?

This is controversial. Because some centres do not operate unless there is neurological deficit or progressive neurological deficits, some may offer surgery before any symptoms develop. Both approaches have advantages and disadvantages. Some would prefer to operate at the earliest sign of neurological deficit. The patient would need to be seen regularly in the clinic and her parents would need to be educated on this.

Case 8

A 40-year-old man presents 3 weeks after a motor vehicle accident with a facial injury and unilateral red eye.

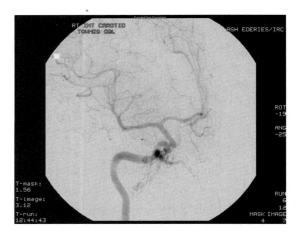

What are the possibilities?

- Carotid-cavernous fistula (CCF) with chemosis and ophthalmoplegia. Examine for bruit, pulsatile exophthalmos and increased intraocular pressure.
- Ocular injury and infection.
- Sinusitis and ophthalmitis.

Describe the findings seen in the image.

This digital subtraction angiogram (DSA) carotid injection image demonstrates dilatation of the superior ophthalmic vein and coil embolization.

How do you classify this condition?

Barrow classification for CCF:

A. Direct high-flow shunt between the internal carotid artery (ICA) and cavernous sinus. Often develops from ruptured cavernous ICA aneurysm.

B. Indirect low-flow dural shunts between meningeal branches of the ICA and the cavernous sinus.

C. Indirect low-flow dural shunts between meningeal branches of the external carotid artery (ECA) and the cavernous sinus.

D. Indirect low-flow dural shunts between meningeal branches of both the ICA and ECA and the cavernous sinus.

What are the factors that would influence your management of this patient?

- High flow.
- Increased intraocular pressure.
- Symptomatic visual deterioration.
- Progressive proptosis.
- On DSA, cortical venous filling.
- Intractable bruit.

What could be performed?

Attempt a coil embolization. The coils could be placed on the feeding artery and/or in the draining superior ophthalmic vein itself.

Following successful treatment, the patient presents later with postural headaches. What could have been the cause?

His headaches could be attributed to CSF rhinorrhea causing low pressure headaches associated with the original injury. In addition, other causes include autonomic dysregulations secondary to hypothalamic injury and hypotension.

How would you investigate a patient with CSF rhinorrhea?

Obtain history: e.g. nasal discharge, 'salty water in the throat', headache that is worse on standing and improves on lying down.

Clinical examination: demonstrate the reservoir sign.

Investigations of the fluid:
- Glucose dipstick test.
- Beta-2 transferrin, a specific marker of CSF.
- Ring or halo sign (less reliable).
- Tau protein.

If the history of low pressure headache is typical and no CSF rhinorrhea is identified, what would your management be?

Investigate for leaking CSF along the neuroaxis with a fine-slice CT scan/CT myelography. I would consider the option of ear, nose, and throat assessment for nasoendoscopy with fluorescein dye.

Reference

Barrow DL, Spector RH, Braun IF, et al. Classification and treatment of spontaneous carotid-cavernous fistulas. *J Neurosurg* 1985: 62: 248–256.

Case 9

A baby is brought to the emergency department by her mother after a fall that occurred 3 days ago. There was a large swelling over the vertex.

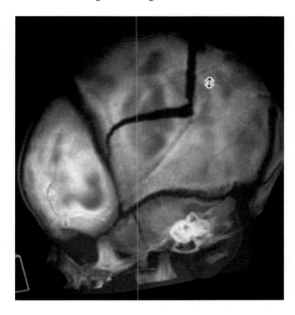

Could you identify the normal and abnormal structures?

Describe the fracture, sutures and vascular markings.

The fracture is more radiolucent than the other sutures, has no serration along its edges, and is blind ending. At the blind end, it is more tapered than at the sutural or proximal end. Vascular markings are less straight and have branches.

Upon stabilization and admission, please state the key steps involved in the patient's management. What other investigations may be necessary?

- Neurological monitoring.
- Activation of the hospital's child protection team. Non-accidental injury (NAI) must be assumed in all such cases.
- CT scan to exclude a chronic subdural haematoma (may not be performed if the child is stable).
- Ophthalmic review for retinal haemorrhage.
- Skeletal survey for old healed fractures.

How would you clinically assess her for increasing ICP?

- Consciousness level (GCS).
- Anterior fontanelle pressure.
- Head circumference.
- Measuring the height at which the fontanelle begins to sink (crude estimate).

Her CT head scan demonstrates a small haematoma deep to the fracture. How would you manage this?

At this stage, the patient would be managed conservatively because the GCS remains stable. There is significant risk of haemorrhage from surgery, particularly bleeding from the superior sagittal sinus.

The mother is a Jehovah's witness who does not agree to blood product transfusion for her child during surgery. How would you take this forward?

If the child requires surgery, I would discuss the options and involve the child protection team, senior colleagues, and hospital solicitors and discuss the options again with the mother. If all fails, I would refer this matter to the court.

The patient was discharged and 6 months later presents with progressively enlarged swelling over the vertex. What could this be?

Leptomeningeal cyst (growing fracture).

Case 10

A 45-year-old woman was brought to the emergency department in a state of stupor after 4 days of neck pain.

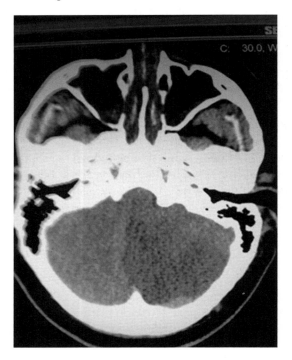

What is the most likely diagnosis?

Left-sided cerebellar infarction with obliteration of the fourth ventricle. I would also consider cerebellar metastasis with surrounding oedema.

What other images would you like to see?

MRI scan with contrast and DWI (including the supratentorial compartment to assess for hydrocephalus) and CTA scan.

What would be your immediate management?

I would have a brief discussion with the family for history and assess the overall condition of the patient. In the meantime I would prepare the patient for surgery. If the patient has gross hydrocephalus, I would insert an EVD followed by wide suboccipital craniectomy and foramen magnum decompression.

The patient recovers well following surgery with a GCS of 14 (E4V4M6). She was noted to have a left-sided partial ptosis and unequal pupils. What could have been the cause?

This could be secondary to disruption of the sympathetic flow secondary to Wallenberg syndrome. I would also like to know from the patient's history if this was congenital or pre-existing.

The neurologist is keen to start the patient on anticoagulants as soon as possible. When would you consider this safe?

Provided there is no contraindication such as expanding haematoma, anticoagulation may be commenced. However, you must balance the benefits and potential risks (including bleeding). A further discussion with the family is recommended.

Case 11

A 46-year-old farmer presents with progressive spastic paraparesis.

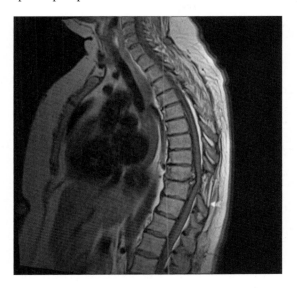

Please describe the MRI scan.

This sagittal T1-weighted MRI scan of the thoracic spine demonstrates a disc bulge in the midthoracic region with spinal cord compression. There is evidence of a previous thoracic decompression.

What will be the next ideal imaging modality to assist you with your surgical planning?

A thoracic CT scan.

Please describe the CT scans below.

Sagittal and axial views of the thoracic CT scan demonstrate a large calcified disc bulge with significant narrowing of the spinal canal.

What are the surgical options?

Two approaches are available here. If the cardiothoracic surgeons are available, my preferred option will be for a right-sided transthoracic approach. If they are not available, I could consider a right-sided costotransversectomy.

What particular care do you have to take while performing the surgery?

Ensure an adequate view of the spinal cord and preserve the artery of Adamkiewicz. In 75% of cases, this artery originates on the left side of the aorta between the T8 and L1 vertebral segments.

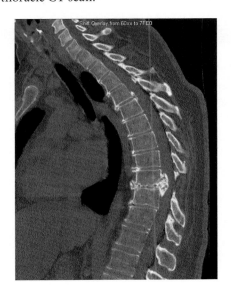

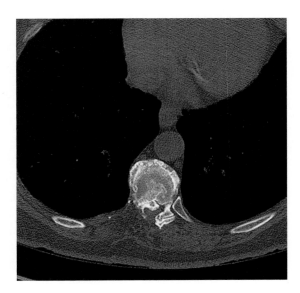

Case 12

A 36-year-old carpenter presents with left-sided brachalgia radiating to his middle finger.

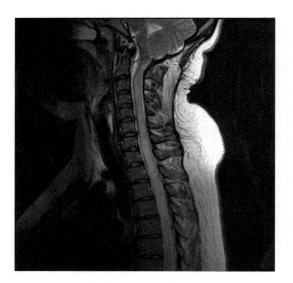

Describe what you see on this image.

Sagittal T2-weighted MRI scan of cervical spine demonstrates multilevel minor cervical disc bulges at C5. There is also a large septated syrinx which extends from the cervico-medullary junction to T6, associated with a type I Chiari malformation.

What operation would you offer this man?

I do not think I have adequate information to decide the best surgical option here. The patient's MRI scan demonstrates multiple abnormalities. May I please ask for further available images?

Describe what you see on the images below.

There is a left-sided C6/7 disc bulge compressing the exiting C7 nerve root, which would correspond to the patient's current symptoms.

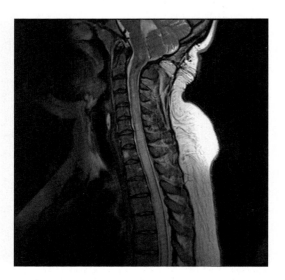

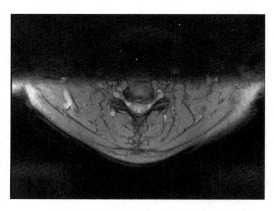

What would you offer him now?

Anterior cervical discectomy and fusion (ACDF), level C6/7.

Case 13

A 56-year-old overweight man woke up with bilateral paraesthesia and weakness (with a left-sided predominance). He has difficulty walking.

How would you manage this patient?

I would take a detailed history and examine the patient to identify the nature of the problem. The sudden nature of his symptoms points to a vascular event. However I could not rule out a spinal pathology because he reports bilateral symptoms involving both upper and lower limbs.

How would you investigate him?

My investigations would include bedside tests (including BP, urinary dipstick and blood glucose measurement) and radiological imaging (CT head scan and spinal MRI scan).

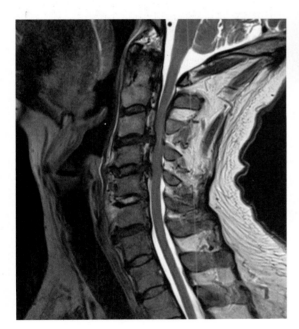

Please describe the spinal MRI scan. All the other tests were normal, including a CT head scan.

Sagittal T2-weighted spinal MRI demonstrates a multilevel disc osteophyte complex with significant spinal cord compression and signal change within the spinal cord.

What would be the next useful investigation?

Cervical CT scan.

Following are the cervical CT images. What is the diagnosis?

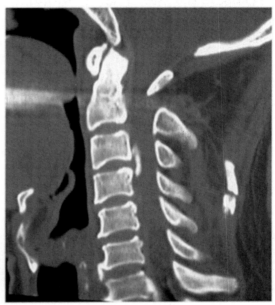

Ossification of posterior longitudinal ligament (OPLL).

How would you manage this condition?

My preferred option would be a posterior cervical decompression; however, because of the loss of cervical lordosis, this may not be effective. Moreover, an anterior cervical decompression could be offered. In addition, I could offer a C3/4 corpectomy (e.g. the worst affected level). A corpectomy may be difficult because the patient is overweight and may have a short neck.

Case 14

A 40-year-old woman presents with pain and numbness in her hands.

(a)

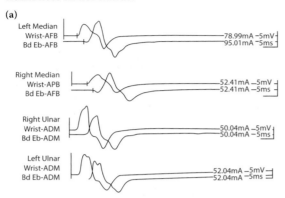

What is the investigation shown in (a), above, and (b), below? Please explain.

The investigation shows median and ulnar nerve conduction studies. The median sensory studies show prolonged sensory latencies of 4.1 ms and 3.5 ms in the right and left hand, respectively. Normal sensory latency is 3.0 ms. There is marked reduction in sensory nerve action potential (SNAP) amplitudes.

What is the diagnosis?

Bilateral carpal tunnel syndrome.

Tips: A quick guide to nerve conduction studies for a neurosurgeon is shown in the following images.

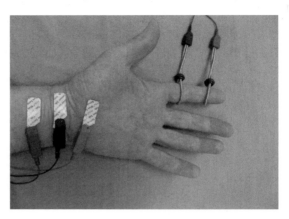

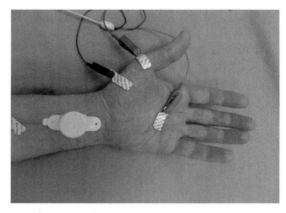

(b)

MNCV Data	Latency (ms)	Amplitude (mv)	CV (m/sec)	Amp %
R Median				
Wrist-APB	4.8	2.9	135.3	89
BE- wrist	6.5	5.5		
	N: ≤ 4ms	N: ≥ 4mv		
L Median				
Wrist-APB	4.5	3.8	115.0	74
BE- wrist	6.5	6.7		
R Ulnar	2.3	10.2		
Wrist-ADM	5.4	7.5	71	−26
BE-wrist	N: ≤ 2ms	N: ≥ 6mv		
L Ulnar				
Wrist ADM	2.2	9.9	65.7	−15
BE-wrist	5.7	8.4		

Sensory, motor or mixed nerves can be studied. Pairs of electrodes are used – one to initiate the impulse and the other to record the response farther along the path of the nerve – for example, distally within the innervated muscle for motor nerves or proximally along sensory nerves. For motor nerves, a depolarizing square wave current is applied to the peripheral nerve to produce a compound muscle action potential (CMAP) due to summation of the activated muscle fibres. In sensory nerves, a propagated SNAP is created in a similar manner.

The parameters obtained and used for interpretation include the following:

- Amplitude – from baseline to peak (reflects the number of conducting fibres and is reduced in axonal loss).
- Latency (ms) – from stimulus to onset of evoked response.
- Duration of response (ms).
- Conduction velocity (m/s) – calculated from the distance between stimulation and recording electrodes.

- Points, divided by latency (reflects integrity of the myelin sheath that are important for impulse conduction and is reduced in demyelinating processes).

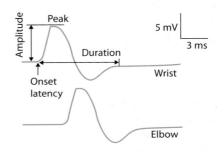

A summary of typical carpal tunnel syndrome follows.

Severity of carpal tunnel	Sensory nerve action potential	Compound motor action potential	Needle EMG activity
Mild	Prolonged latency	Normal	Normal
Moderate	Prolonged latency and decreased amplitude	Prolonged latency	Normal
Severe	Absent	Prolonged latency and decreased amplitude	Abnormal activity

References

DeLisa JA, Gans BM. *Physical Medicine and Rehabilitation: principles and practice.* 4th ed. Philadelphia: Lippincott Williams & Wilkins; 2005.

Weiss LD, Silver JK, Weiss J. *Easy EMG: a guide to performing nerve conduction studies and electromyography.* Edinburgh, New York: Butterworth-Heinemann; 2004.

Case 15

A 35-year-old woman is brought into the emergency department at 23:00 after a road traffic accident (RTA). She has no neurological deficits.

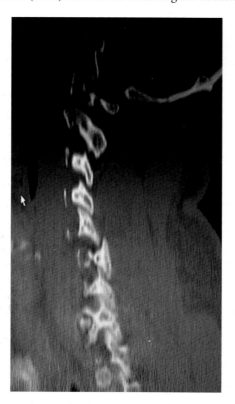

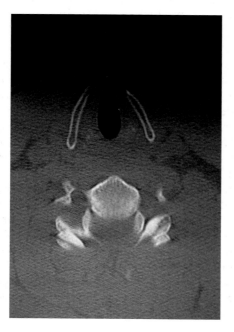

What is the most likely diagnosis?

Unilateral C5/6 locked facet. The risk of neurological compromise in bilateral locked facet is very high although there are intact patients in rare circumstances. If the degree of subluxation exceeds 50 per cent, then it is most probably bilateral locked facet.

Would you request an MRI scan at this stage?

Yes. However, there is no urgency for this. A traumatic disc and haemorrhage have to be ruled out. It is also helpful to know the integrity of spinal ligaments, particularly posterior longitudinal ligaments. Cervical traction should be applied with caution should the MRI scan demonstrate disrupted ligaments.

The patient starts to develop paraparesis of all her limbs to MRC Grade 3/5. What are the options for treatment?

This would be in keeping with cord compression due to locked facet, traumatic disc, haematoma or progressive oedema. Poor resuscitation techniques, patient transfer or cervical immobilization could aggravate neurological injury.

How would MRI help in the surgical planning? Briefly describe the treatment options.

The patient would need stabilization in both anterior and posterior planes. If there is a traumatic disc, then an anterior discectomy needs to be performed before turning over the patient and reducing the subluxation posteriorly and then turning her again for anterior stabilization. Alternatively, a posterior stabilization under cervical traction could be performed. The perched superior facet could be drilled and reduced. Posterior instrumentation could be followed by anterior stabilization. The use of intraoperative image intensifiers or such modalities is vital. The level of cervical traction would largely depend on the cervical level and condition of spinal ligaments. The anaesthetist needs to be aware of this because increasing muscle relaxation reduces the amount of cervical traction.

The other option is prolonged cervical immobilization if there are strong reasons for a patient who is unsuitable for surgery. However this has risks associated with prolonged hospital stay and immobilization. The rate of fusion among patients varies with unilateral or bilateral locked facet (only about 20% in the latter), ligamental integrity, age, smoking status, presence of any comorbidities and patient compliance.

While waiting, the patient develops a headache and progressive drop in consciousness. How would you investigate this?

The management would still follow the advanced trauma life support (ATLS) principles of maintaining airway, breathing and circulation. This should be followed by a detailed examination to identify a localizing sign such as papillary changes or hemiparesis. Then the subsequent management would depend on the cause. The possibilities include the following:

1. The patient's pre-existing condition needs to be taken into account. This includes diabetes mellitus (risk of hypoglycaemia), use of drugs and substances (overdosage or withdrawal), alcoholism (withdrawal, seizures) and overdose of opiates.

2. In the trauma setting, spinal injury and an associated head injury occur in about 20% of patients, and some of them can be missed during the primary survey. Expanding intracranial haematoma, particularly extradural haematoma, can be missed as a result of the lucid interval. Other lesions could be subdural haematoma, contusion and associated seizure.

3. The risk of vertebral artery dissection should be considered in patients with spinal injury that involves the foramen transversarium. The patient could develop cerebellar or brainstem infarction and oedema of the posterior fossa structures. This would result in an acute obstructive hydrocephalus. The patient would typically present with severe headache and reducing level of consciousness.

4. The patient may have developed spinal cord compression at this stage as a result of instability, and this could potentially result in spinal shock and altered sensorium. Reassessment of her limbs and anal tone is important at this stage. In males, priapism can be seen. This can also develop iatrogenically during transfer or turning without adequate cervical spine immobilization. Other possibilities are expanding haematoma with the spinal canal, traumatic intervertebral disc and spinal artery compression.

5. Hypovolaemic shock could present in altered sensorium and be misleading. An abdominal examination and Focussed Assessment with Sonography in Trauma (FAST) would rapidly assess for gross intra-abdominal bleeding. However, guided by the patient's haemodynamic status, a chest, abdomen and pelvis CT scan should be requested if there is a suggestion of solid organ injury and evidence of haemorrhage.

If the patient presented with complete non-sacral-sparing paraplegia, how would you manage her?

In complete spinal cord injury the chance of recovery is very small and there is no evidence to suggest that urgent surgical intervention would improve outcome. The patient requires spinal care including adequate hydration, blood pressure maintenance (MAP of 90 mmHg) and catheterization. I would ensure the patient is nursed on a spinal bed and is given prophylaxis for stress ulcers. I would spend time explaining and counselling the patient and family about her condition. This is crucial to minimize secondary injury to the cord, which could influence her upper limb function in particular. There is a role for decompression and fusion of the fracture, mainly for nursing and mobility purposes, and this could be done on a scheduled list with a trained theatre team on spinal care. This would reduce the chances of developing pressure ulcers and improve the outlook for the patient.

Another scenario: During an outpatient clinic, you review the same patient following her road traffic accident with similar CT images. How would you manage her?

In this case, I would explain to her that she has a potentially unstable injury and would try to convince her to be admitted. The options are cervical traction with Gardner-Wells tongs or surgery.

I would provide analgesics and apply gentle cervical traction, gradually increasing the weight. The ideal weight is 5 lb per level of cervical vertebrae; therefore, in her case, this would be 25lb to 30lb. I would perform serial X-rays before and after the weights are applied. Closed neurological monitoring is needed, particularly for numbness or weakness of limbs. Once the spine is reduced, a halo could be applied to maintain the reduction; this has to be confirmed with X-rays. If this fails, she can be recommended for early surgery during the same admission. Surgery can be performed with sliding traction to assist reduction.

Case 16

A 33-year-old man is scheduled for a left selective amygdalohippocampectomy (SAH). A digital subtraction angiography (DSA) was performed for an amytal test.

What is an amytal (Wada) test and what does it assess?

A Wada test involves infusion of amytal sodium to create a temporary chemical dysfunction of either hemisphere. It is usually performed as a preoperative investigation for lateralizing speech and memory in temporal lobe resection for epilepsy.

What is the abnormality shown, and is it safe to continue with the amytal test? What precaution needs to be taken?

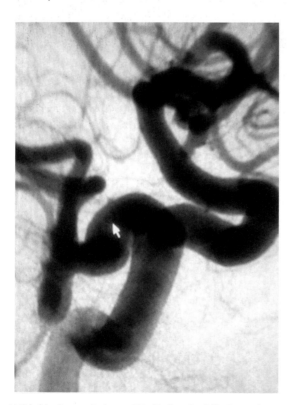

With kind permission of Dr Rufus Corkill, Consultant Radiologist, John Radcliffe Hospital, Oxford.

The angiogram shows a carotid DSA. There is an abnormal communication between the ICA and basilar artery before the carotid siphon. This could be a persistent trigeminal artery. Amytal testing would be risky in this patient because this could cause temporary dysfunction of the brainstem and cardiorespiratory arrest. However, amytal injected distal to the artery would be safe.

What adjuncts could be done to investigate a patient going for temporal lobe resection in epilepsy surgery?

Functional MRI scan and neuropsychological assessment.

Investigations revealed that he has bilateral mesial temporal lobe epilepsy (MTLE) and is not a suitable candidate for surgical resection. How would you manage him?

I would discuss the patient with the epileptologist in regard to medical management. Alternatively, a vagal nerve stimulator could be offered.

Case 17

A 29-year-old woman with a body mass index (BMI) of 56 presented via an ophthalmologist with a 3-month history of increasing headache, left facial numbness, diplopia and papilloedema. She undergoes an MRI scan.

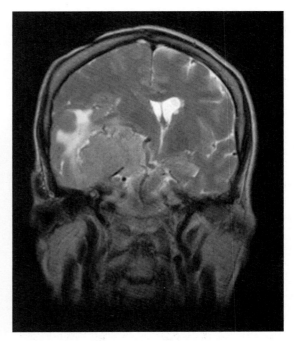

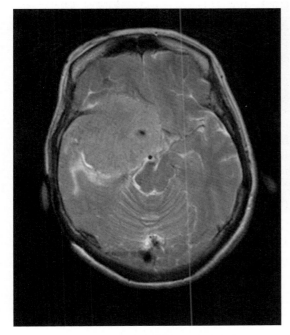

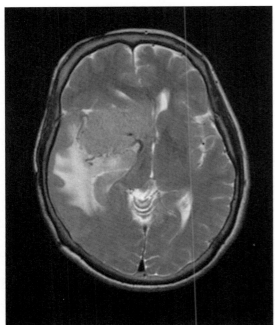

How would you manage this patient?

Her MRI head scan demonstrates a very large extra-axial avidly enhancing mass straddling and arising from the right sphenoid ridge. There is associated mass effect, signal change and subfalcine herniation. Further investigations are warranted:

- DSA +/- embolization (one should be prepared to take the patient to surgery following embolization if there is a sudden neurological deterioration of the condition as a result of post-embolization swelling).
- CT angiogram to assess the tumour's vascularity.

What are your differential diagnoses?

- Large sphenoid wing meningioma.
- Hemangiopericytoma.
- Solitary metastatic tumour.

She went on to have resection of the tumour. What does the following slide demonstrate?

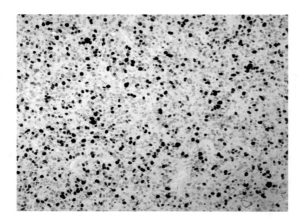

This is a Ki-67 stained slide showing moderately high proliferative index.

Ki-67 is a cellular marker for proliferation. It is strictly associated with cell proliferation. Ki-67 protein is present during all active phases of the cell cycle (G_1, S, G_2, and mitosis) but is absent from resting cells (G_0).

Small areas of the tumour show the following characteristic features. What is this?

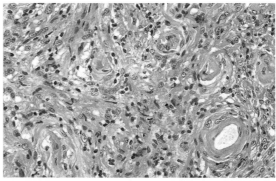

Meningothelial whorl pattern in an underlying meningioma.

What is the diagnosis?

Atypical meningioma.

Are there any features on the previous MRI scan to support this diagnosis?

Yes, the lobulated appearance of the lesion.

6

The viva: the non-operative clinical practice of neurosurgery

The non-operative clinical practice of neurosurgery is an important aspect of the oral and clinical examination. The majority of candidates spend an enormous effort memorizing precise values, ranges and units for certain neurosurgical conditions. Although specific figures are important, the emphasis of the examination is to demonstrate your understanding of the basic principles.

For example: 'A positron emission tomography (PET) scan is a nuclear medical imaging technique that produces three-dimensional images. The technique involves the administration of a metabolically active, radioactive tracer that spontaneously decays to release positrons. These positrons travel a short distance into adjacent tissue where they are annihilated by reacting with electrons. This annihilation reaction results in the release of paired, high-energy photons that travel in opposite directions from each other and are detected by a PET scanner. PET imaging has potential benefits in neuroncology, ischaemic cerebrovascular disease and epilepsy. Limitations of this test include availability and the short half-life of isotopes. For example, the test may be challenging in the evaluation of an ictal foci in epilepsy. In these cases, a single-photon emission computed tomography (SPECT) scan is more sensitive.'

Apply your basic knowledge to the real solutions. Occasionally, you may be asked to talk about a broad topic (however, most examiners would tend to avoid this). In this overwhelming situation, do not rush to mention a specific point because this may generate questions regarding this point and only results in an incomplete answer. It is best to give a 'frame' or subdivision to the topic, and then proceed to describe each point. It is recommended to begin the discussion around the most relevant or common topic.

Top tip: **'Define, Classify, Amplify'.**

For example, if the examiner asks you to discuss the principles of 'neuroprotection', it is not advised to start with one potential treatment: hypothermia. You would then be expected to know that hypothermia results in a reduction in cerebral metabolism ($CMRO_2$) by approximately 7 per cent per 1°C. This also leads to less oxygen and glucose consumption.

The authors recommend the following structured answer:

Define: 'Neuroprotection' refers to the preservation of neuronal structure and function. Neuroprotection aims to prevent or slow disease progression and secondary injuries by halting or at least slowing the loss of neurons.

Classify: Common mechanisms of neuronal loss include increased levels in oxidative stress, mitochondrial dysfunction, excitotoxicity, inflammatory changes, iron accumulation, and protein aggregation. Common neuroprotective treatments include glutamate antagonists and antioxidants, which aim to limit excitotoxicity and oxidative stress respectively.

Amplify: Other treatments include caspase inhibitors, trophic factors, anti-protein aggregation agents and hypothermia.

The following key topics are discussed:

1. Neuro-critical care: management of raised intracranial pressure (ICP).
2. Seizures.
3. Hyponatraemia.
4. Diabetes insipidus.
5. Brainstem testing.
6. Back pain and cauda equina syndrome.
7. Pain pathways.
8. Neuropharmacology.
9. Informed consent.
10. Management of common neurosurgical conditions.

These key topics are not a comprehensive list. The examiners will examine your logical arguments regarding controversial points. Samples of these debates are mentioned at the end of each topic (e.g. evidence of outcome measures for ICP monitoring, the overlap between syndrome of inappropriate antidiuretic hormone secretion [SIADH] and cerebral salt wasting [CSW], and screening for aneurysms).

Case scenarios

Case 1: Neuro-critical care: management of raised intracranial pressure

An 18-year-old man is involved in a high-speed traffic accident. At the scene, his Glasgow Coma Score (GCS) is 6. On arrival at the trauma centre, he is intubated and a computed tomography (CT) scan is performed. He has diffuse cerebral oedema with effacement of the sulci. He is being monitored in the Surgical Intensive Care Unit.

How do you assess for adequate blood supply to the brain?

- Cerebral blood flow (CBF): blood supply per unit area of cerebral tissue per unit time.
- Directly proportional to volume of blood, but inversely related to vascular resistance.
- CBF = cerebral perfusion pressure (CPP)/cerebral vascular resistance (CVR).
  - Normal: 55–60 mL per 100 g per minute.
  - Hyperaemia: CBF in excess of 55–60 mL per 100 g per minute.
  - Ischemia: CBF below 18–20 mL per 100 g per minute.
  - Tissue death: CBF below 8–10 mL per 100 g per minute.

How do you control cerebral blood flow?

- Modulate factors affecting the cerebral perfusion pressure (CPP = mean arterial pressure [MAP] – intracranial pressure [ICP]).
- Modulate factors affecting cerebral vascular resistance (CVR).

CVR is controlled by four major mechanisms:
1. Metabolic control.
2. Pressure autoregulation.
3. Chemical control (by arterial pCO_2 and pO_2).
4. Neural control.

What is autoregulation? Describe the mechanisms.

- Autoregulation is the intrinsic ability of brain vasculature to maintain constant CBF over a wide range of blood pressures.
- Vessel calibre changes are mediated by interplay between myogenic and metabolic mechanisms.
- Autoregulation can be modulated by the following:
  - Sympathetic nervous activity.
  - Renin–angiotensin system.
  - Arterial carbon dioxide tension.

What is ICP?

Intracranial pressure is the pressure exerted by the intracranial content. The Monro–Kellie hypothesis states that the sum of the intracranial volumes of blood (CBV), brain, cerebrospinal fluid (CSF), and other components (tumour, haematoma) is constant, and that an increase in any one of these must be offset by an equal decrease in another, or else the overall pressure will rise. These volumes are contained in a rigid fixed skull. The pressure is distributed evenly throughout the intracranial cavity (Figure 6.1).

What is a normal ICP waveform?

Normal ICP waves usually consist of three arterial components superimposed on the respiratory rhythm (Figure 6.2).

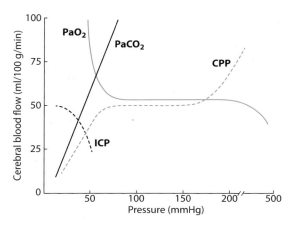

Figure 6.1 Intracranial pressure.

Percussion wave: arterial pressure transmitted from the choroid plexus.
Tidal wave: ventricular relaxation.
Dicrotic wave: closure of aortic valve.
Compliance: dV/dP (Figure 6.3).

What are pathological ICP waveforms?

Lundberg A waves (plateau waves)

- These indicate an abrupt increase in ICP ≥ 50 mm Hg for 5–20 minutes followed by rapid fall in ICP.
- The plateau wave represents a transient increased CBV, possibly secondary to CO_2 retention.

Lundberg B waves (pressure pulses)

- Amplitude of 10–20 mmHg with rhythmic variation 0.5–2 min.

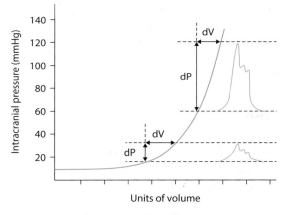

Figure 6.3 Compliance.

Lundberg C waves

- Frequency of 4–8/min. Low amplitude C wave may be seen in a normal ICP waveform. High amplitude C wave may be pre-terminal, and may sometimes be seen on top of plateau waves.

How do you manage increased ICP in a head injury patient?

1. Advanced trauma life support (ATLS).
   - ABCDE (Airway maintenance and cervical spine protection, breathing and ventilation, circulation with haemorrhage control, disability and neurological assessment, exposure and environmental control).

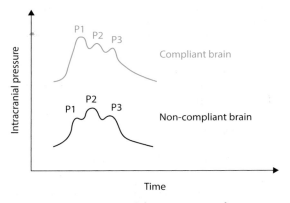

Figure 6.2 Intracranial pressure waveform.

2. Physiological.
   - Elevate the head (30–40°); this will reduce venous congestion.
   - Relieve jugular compression by straightening the neck, loosening bandages.
   - Avoid hypoxia and hypercarbia.
   - Maintain mean arterial blood pressure (MAP) >90 mmHg.
   - Correct electrolyte balance (hyponatraemia, hyperglycaemia).
3. Control seizures with anticonvulsants.
4. Pharmacological.
   - Intubation, ventilation and sedation.
   - Adequate analgesia.
   - Osmotic diuretics: mannitol.
   - Barbiturates as needed to obtain burst suppression on electroencephalography (EEG).
5. Surgical.
   - CSF drainage procedure (external ventricular drain [EVD]).
   - Removal of causes of increased ICP (space-occupying lesion).
   - Decompressive craniectomy.

What is the blood–brain barrier?

The blood-brain barrier (BBB) is a physiological barrier between the brain parenchyma and systemic circulation. Unlike the somatic capillaries, endothelial fenestration is absent in brain capillaries. The BBB is composed of capillary endothelial tight junctions, pinocytic activity in endothelial cells and astrocytic foot processes. Movement across the BBB occurs by diffusion, carrier-mediated transport or active transport. The BBB is absent in the following areas:

> Area postrema.
> Median eminence of the hypothalamus.
> Neurohypophysis.
> Organum vasculosum (lamina terminalis).
> Pineal gland.
> Subcommissural organ.
> Subfornical organ.

The permeability across the BBB differs.

> Highly permeable: water, CO_2, O_2, lipid-soluble (ethanol, barbiturates).
> Slightly permeable: ions (sodium, potassium and chloride).
> Impermeable: plasma proteins, protein-bound molecules, large organic molecules and L-glucose.

What are the four types of cerebral oedema? Which one is associated with severe head injuries?

1. Vasogenic: The BBB is disrupted. Protein leaks out of the vascular system and the extracellular space expands. Leakage of plasma content into the intracellular space. Vasogenic oedema responses to corticosteroids (dexamethasone). Example: brain tumour, infection, trauma.
2. Osmotic: Plasma dilution decreases serum osmolality, resulting in a higher osmolality in the brain compared to the serum. This creates an abnormal pressure gradient and movement of water into the brain, which can cause swelling. Example: hyponatraemia, SIADH.
3. Interstitial: There is rupture of the CSF–brain barrier. This results in trans-ependymal flow of CSF, causing CSF to penetrate the brain and spread to the extracellular spaces and the white matter. Example: obstructive hydrocephalus.
4. Cytotoxic: the BBB remains intact. There is disruption in cellular metabolism that impairs functioning of the sodium and potassium pump in the glial cell membrane, leading to cellular retention of sodium and water. Swollen astrocytes occur in grey and white matter. Example: severe head injury.

Potential debates for discussion

> Does ICP monitoring influence outcome in head injuries?
> Does ICP management influence outcome in head injuries?
> ICP management in paediatric head injuries.
> Overlap and differentiation between different types of brain oedema.

Case 2: Seizures

A 52-year-old woman presents with a history of longstanding right-sided headaches associated with olfactory aura. Her MRI scan demonstrates a right-sided sphenoid wing meningioma.

What are seizures?

Seizures are abnormal paroxysmal cerebral neuronal discharges resulting in psychomotor and sensory abnormalities. They can be classified based on whether the source of the seizure within the brain is localized (partial) or distributed (generalized).

Partial seizures: one hemisphere involved at the onset.

1. Simple partial seizures.
   - Motor.
   - Sensory.
2. Complex partial.
3. Complex partial with secondary generalization.

Generalized seizures: bilaterally symmetrical and synchronous involving both hemispheres at the onset (with no local onset) and associated with a documented loss of conscience.

1. Absence.
2. Tonic.
3. Clonic.
4. Generalized tonic clonic (GTC).
5. Atonic.
6. Myoclonic.

How do you classify seizures?

Symptomatic: seizures of known aetiology (cerebrovascular accident [CVA], trauma, tumour, vascular causes, metabolic causes or infection).

Idiopathic: no underlying cause identified (juvenile myoclonic epilepsy).

Cryptogenic: seizures presumed to be symptomatic, but with unknown aetiology (West syndrome, Lennox–Gastaut syndrome).

Special syndromes: situational-related seizures (febrile seizures, alcohol withdrawal).

How do you investigate seizures?

- History and examination (vitally important to rule out the abovementioned causes).
- Standard blood tests.
- EEG.
- MRI scan.

How do you manage seizures?

Remove any reversible causes.

Identify factors that lower seizure threshold (sleep deprivation, hyperventilation, photic stimulation, infection, electrolyte disturbance, head injury, and cerebral ischaemia).

The UK National Institute for Health and Care Excellence (NICE) Guidelines (CG137) recommend the following:

- Tonic clonic or generalized seizures:
  - First-line treatment in patients with newly diagnosed GTC seizures includes the following:
    - Sodium valproate.
    - Lamotrigine – if sodium valproate is unsuitable.
  - Adjunctive treatment in patient with GTC seizures includes the following:
    - Clobazam, lamotrigine, levetiracetam, sodium valproate or topiramate if first-line treatments are ineffective or not tolerated.
  - In the presence of absence or myoclonic seizures, or if juvenile myoclonic epilepsy (JME) is suspected, do not give carbamazepine, gabapentin, oxcarbazepine, phenytoin, pregabalin, tiagabine or vigabatrin.
- Focal seizures:
  - First-line treatment in patient with newly diagnosed focal seizures includes the following:
    - Carbamazepine or lamotrigine
    - Levetiracetam, oxcarbazepine or sodium valproate (teratogenic risks) – if carbamazepine and lamotrigine are unsuitable or not tolerated.
  - If the first antiepileptic drug (AED) tried is ineffective, offer an alternative from these five AEDs. Adjunctive treatment should be considered if a second well-tolerated AED is ineffective.

continued

- Adjunctive treatment in patient with refractory focal seizures includes the following:
  - Carbamazepine, clobazam, gabapentin, lamotrigine, levetiracetam oxcarbazepine, sodium valproate or topiramate as adjunctive treatment in patient with focal seizures if first-line treatments are ineffective or not tolerated.
- Petit mal or absence seizures: treatment with ethosuximide, lamotrigine or sodium valproate.
- Myoclonic seizures: sodium valproate.
- Infantile spasms: vigabatrin.

Regarding the newer AEDs, National Institute for Health and Care Excellence (NICE) recommends that newer AEDs, gabapentin, lamotrigine, levetiracetam, oxcarbazepine, tiagabine, topiramate and vigabatrin, within their licensed indications, are recommended for the management of epilepsy in adults who have not benefited from treatment with the older antiepileptic drugs such as carbamazepine or sodium valproate, or for whom the older antiepileptic drugs are unsuitable. Reasons for unsuitability include the following:

- There are contraindications to the drugs.
- They could interact with other drugs the person is taking (notably oral contraceptives).
- They are already known to be poorly tolerated by the individual.
- The person is a woman of childbearing potential.

Which anticonvulsants are recommended in pregnancy?

In general, the risk of seizures (including maternal and fetal hypoxia and acidosis) outweighs the potential teratogenic risk of most anticonvulsants.

- Proper seizure control is the primary goal in treating pregnant women.
- Monotherapy is recommended over polytherapy.
- The lowest effective dose of carbamazepine is recommended.

Reference

National Clinical Guideline Centre (NCGC). *The epilepsies: the diagnosis and management of the epilepsies in adults and children in primary and secondary care.* 2012. Commissioned by the National Institute for Health and Clinical Excellence.
(Please refer to your National Guidelines because they are subject to change.)

Potential debates for discussion

Identification of pseudoseizures.
Definition of status epilepticus.
Monitoring for seizure activity in the ventilated patient.

Case 3: Hyponatraemia

An 83-year-old woman underwent a burr-hole evacuation of a chronic subdural haematoma. On day 3, she becomes confused and agitated. She is diagnosed with hyponatraemia with a serum sodium of 121. The trend demonstrates progressive hyponatraemia.

Management of syndrome of inappropriate antidiuretic hormone secretion (SIADH)/cerebral salt-wasting syndrome (CSW).

What are the causes of hyponatraemia?

- Hypovolaemic hyponatraemia: sodium and free water loss with inappropriate hypotonic fluid replacement.
  - CSW: severe head injury, aneurysmal subarachnoid haemorrhage, and subdural haematoma.
  - Gastrointestinal loss: vomiting and diarrhoea.
  - Excessive sweating.
  - Third space pooling: peritonitis, pancreatitis, burns.
  - Renal insufficiency.
  - Prolonged exercise in a hot environment.
- Euvolemic hyponatraemia: normal sodium stores and total body excess free water.
  - Psychogenic polydipsia.
  - Hypotonic intravenous or irrigation fluids.
- Hypervolaemic hyponatraemia: inappropriate increase in sodium stores.
  - **SIADH.**
  - **Medication** (thiazide diuretics, carbamazepine, acetazolamide, angiotensin-converting enzyme inhibitors, gabapentin, haloperidol, heparin, loop diuretics, nimodipine, proton pump inhibitors, selective serotonin reuptake inhibitors).
  - Hepatic cirrhosis.
  - Congestive heart failure.
  - Nephrotic syndrome.
  - Hypothyroidism.
- Cortisol deficiency.

How would you investigate this patient's hyponatraemia?

- Take a comprehensive history and examine the patient.
- Review fluid balance charts.
- Order blood test (serum and urine sodium and osmolalities, urine specific gravity, serum electrolytes, thyroid function and adrenal function).

How do you make the diagnosis of SIADH?

The diagnosis is based on history, clinical examination and blood and urine results. Patient may present with confusion, lethargy, nausea/vomiting, seizures, coma and possible fluid overload. The diagnostic criteria include hyponatraemia, inappropriately concentrated urine and evidence of renal and adrenal dysfunction.

1. Low serum sodium < 134 mEq/L.
2. Low serum osmolality < 280 mOsm/L.
3. High urinary sodium >18 mEq/L, often 50–150.
4. High ratio of urine:serum osmolality: 1.5–2.1:1.
5. Normal renal and adrenal function.
6. No hypothyroidism.
7. No clinical signs of dehydration or overhydration.

How do you treat SIADH?

- Liaise with endocrinology department.
- If mild and asymptomatic, consider fluid restriction <1 L/day.
- If severe or symptomatic, consider hypertonic saline.
- Correct hyponatraemia slowly (no more than 8–10 mmol/L of sodium per day) to prevent central pontine myelinolysis (CPM).

Biochemical marker	SIADH	CSWS
Intravascular volume status	Normal to high	Low
Serum sodium	Low	Low
Urinary sodium level	High	Very high
Vasopressin level	High	Low
Urine output	Normal or low	High
Serum uric acid level	Low	Low
Initial fractional excretion of urate	High	High
Fractional excretion of urate after correction of hyponatraemia	Normal	High
Urinary osmolality	High	High
Serum osmolality	Low	Low
Blood urea nitrogen/creatinine level	Low to normal	High
Serum potassium level	Normal	Normal to high
Central venous pressure	Normal to high	Low
Pulmonary capillary wedge pressure	Normal to high	Low
Brain natriuretic peptide level	Normal	High
Treatment	Water restriction	Fluids and/or mineralocorticoid

CSWS – Cerebral salt wasting syndrome; SIADH – syndrome of inappropriate antidiuretic hormone.

Case 4: Management of diabetes insipidus

A 43-year-old man underwent an endoscopic endonasal resection of a craniopharyngioma. Post-operatively, the patient is thirsty with a high urine output >300 mL/h.

What is his diagnosis?

Diabetes insipidus (DI) is a result of low circulating levels of antidiuretic hormone (ADH) (or rarely, renal insensitivity secondary to ADH). The insufficiency of ADH results on the excessive renal loss of water and electrolytes. Patients have a high output of dilute urine (<200 mOsm/L or specific gravity <1.003) with normal or high serum osmolality. They often present with a craving for fluids.

DI can be classified into central/neurogenic or nephrogenic DI.

Central/neurogenic DI is caused by hypothalamic-pituitary axis dysfunction.

- Familial (autosomal dominant).
- Idiopathic.
- Posttraumatic (including surgery).
- Tumour (craniopharyngioma, metastasis, lymphoma).
- Granuloma (neurosarcoidosis, histiocytosis).
- Infection (meningitis, encephalitis).
- Autoimmune.
- Vascular (aneurysm, Sheehan's syndrome).

Nephrogenic DI is associated with relative resistance of the kidney to normal or supranormal levels of ADH.

- Familial (X-linked recessive).
- Hypokalemia.
- Hypercalcemia.
- Sjögren's syndrome.
- Drugs: lithium.
- Chronic renal disease.

How do you make the diagnosis?

1. Dilute urine.
   Urine osmolality <200 mOsm/L or specific gravity <1.003.
   Inability to concentrate urine to >300 mOsm/L in the presence of clinical dehydration.
2. Urine output >250 mL/h.
3. Normal or above-normal serum sodium.
4. Normal adrenal function.

What is the triphasic response?

Following transsphenoidal surgery or removal of a craniopharyngioma, central DI results because of injury to the posterior pituitary. Three patterns are seen.

Transient DI: supra-normal urine output and polydipsia that normalizes within 12–36 hours.
Prolonged DI: supra-normal urine output occurring for prolonged periods of time (months) to permanently (years).
Triphasic DI:
  Phase 1: Injury to the pituitary gland reduces ADH levels for 4–5 days, and patients present with polyuria/polydipsia.
  Phase 2: Cell death releases ADH for the next 4–5 days, and there is a transient normalization or even SIADH-like water retention.
  Phase 3: Reduced or absent ADH secretion results in transient or prolonged DI.

How do you manage DI?

If DI is mild and the patient's thirst mechanism is intact, instruct the patient to drink only when thirsty; in this way, patients can usually keep up with their fluid losses. If DI is severe, patients may not be able to take in an adequate intake of fluids to meet their losses. In these cases, desmopressin (DDVAP) can be given by the oral, nasal or intravenous route.

Potential debates for discussion

The overlap between SIADH and CSW.
Switchover phases between CSW and SIADH.
Adipsic DI.

Case 5: Brainstem testing

A 73-year-old man is thrown off his motorbike while driving home. He lost control as a result of bad weather. On arrival at the emergency department, his GCS is 3, and his pupils are fixed and dilated.

What is brainstem death?

Brainstem death is diagnosed by the cessation of function *and* irreversibility of cessation of either the cardiopulmonary system or the entire brain.

What are the brainstem death criteria?

In the UK, the tests should be carried out by two qualified doctors who are competent with the procedure; one of these should be a consultant, and both should have been fully registered with the General Medical Council for at least 5 years. The test must be undertaken by the two doctors and completed successfully on two separate occasions.

Exclusion criteria: reversible causes (e.g. hypothermia, drugs, metabolic and endocrine abnormalities and shock) must be corrected.

Ventilator dependence is confirmed by disconnection for a period to ensure that the medullary respiratory centre is exposed to a powerful hypercapnic drive stimulus ($PaCO_2$ $\geq$6.65 kPa or >60 mmHg).

The prescribed testing is required to be repeated, at an unspecified interval, 'to ensure that there has been no observer error'.

Potential debates for discussion

Role and interpretation of brainstem auditory evoked potentials (BSAEP), transcranial Doppler (TCD) and angiography in brainstem death tests.

Absence of brainstem reflexes	
Absent pupillary light reflex	Pupils are fixed and do not respond to light.
Absent corneal reflexes	
Absent oculovestibular reflex	In a clean and unobstructed ear canal, 20 mL of iced water is irrigated. There should be no eye movement in response to the cold stimulus.
Absent oculocephalic reflex	Sudden rotation of the head from side to side results in a negative doll's eye, in which the eyes would stay fixed in mid-orbit position.
Absent gag and cough reflex	
Apnoea test	The patient is pre-oxygenated with 100% oxygen; the ventilator is turned off and oxygen is given via nasal cannula (6–8 L/minute); blood gases are obtained; when $PaCO_2$ >6.65 kPA or >60 mm Hg, the apnoea test is positive if there is no respiratory effort.
No response to deep central pain	No response to supraorbital painful stimuli.
Observations	Core temperature >32.2°C, SBP $\geq$90 mm Hg.

Case 6: Back pain and cauda equina syndrome

A 32-year-old woman presents with an acute-on-chronic history of lower back pain. After returning from a skiing holiday, she presents with a severe episode of back pain, bilateral weakness in the lower limbs and urinary incontinence.

What are the 'red flags' on clinical history and examination?
Clinical history

- Age >50 years.
- Cancer: history of cancer, unexplained weight loss, pain at multiple sites.
- Night pain (not mechanical in nature).
- Immunosuppression: human immunodeficiency virus (HIV), steroid use, diabetes mellitus (DM), organ transplantation.
- Infection: fever, night sweats, back tenderness, limited range of movement.
- Cauda equina syndrome: sphincter dysfunction, saddle anaesthesia, leg pain, paraesthesia or weakness.
- Trauma: major or minor (osteoporotic patients).
- Intractability.
- Neurological symptoms.

Clinical examination

- Saddle anaesthesia.
- Incontinence.
- Fever >38°C.
- Urinary retention.
- Muscular weakness.
- Bony tenderness (vertebral).
- Limited range of spinal motion.

How do you differentiate between neurogenic and vascular claudication?
Neurogenic claudication

Symptoms.
Leg pain with standing or walking.
Weakness, 'giving way'.
Associated with numbness (dermatomal).
Worse with walking or standing.
Relieved quickly with sitting or bending forward.

Signs.
Normal examination.
The following may be present:
Reduced deep tendon reflexes.
Dermatomal paraesthesia.
Positive straight leg raise test.
Wide-based gait.

Vascular claudication

Symptoms.
Calf pain with walking.
Buttock, thigh pain ± foot pain.
Worse when walking or activity.
Relieved with minutes of rest.
Paraesthesia ± weakness.
Rest pain (advanced).
Signs.
Reduced pulses and bruits.
Skin changes (arterial insufficiency).
Pallor on elevation.
Dusky rubor on dependence (Buerger's).

What is cauda equina syndrome?

Cauda equina syndrome (CES) is a serious neurological condition in which damage to the cauda equina causes loss of function of the lumbar plexus (nerve roots) of the spinal canal below the termination (conus medullaris) of the spinal cord.

What are the most common symptoms and signs of cauda equine syndrome?

- Lower back pain.
- Bilateral sciatica.
- Saddle anaesthesia.
- Motor weakness of the lower extremities.
- Rectal and bladder sphincter dysfunction.
- Urinary dysfunction (retention and incontinence).
- Reduced anal sphincter tone.

Where are the bladder control centres?

There are three main centres:

- Frontal lobe: anteromedial frontal lobe and corpus callosum, which are involved in conscious inhibition.

- Nucleus locus coeruleus of the pons: synchronizes the detrusor muscle contraction with relaxation of the urethral sphincter. It regulates both sympathetic and parasympathetic responses.
- Sacral centre: the reflex centre.

Describe the physiology of bladder control

The lower urinary tract is innervated by three principal sets of peripheral nerves involving the parasympathetic, sympathetic, and somatic nervous systems from three major nerves, namely the pelvic, hypogastric and pudendal nerves, respectively.

Motor control
Autonomic (involuntary)

Parasympathetic control: S2-S4 (cell bodies in intermediolateral column of grey matter of the spinal cord) to the pelvic splanchnic nerves (nervi erigentes) to the ganglia in the muscle wall (detrusor muscles).

Sympathetic control: T12-L2 (cell bodies in intermediolateral column of grey matter of the spinal cord) to the pre-ganglionic axons to inferior mesenteric ganglion to the inferior hypogastric plexus to the bladder wall and internal sphincters.

Somatic control (voluntary)

Control originates from the frontal lobe and descends along the pyramidal tract into the pudendal nerve to innervate the external sphincters.

Sensory control

Bladder distension is detected by sensory stretch receptors on the muscle wall. An action potential is generated along the first order sensory neurons, which travel along the autonomic fibres (via pelvic, hypogastric and pudendal nerves) to the conus medullaris and then ascend primarily in the spinothalamic tract.

How should this patient be managed?

She requires an urgent operation (e.g. microdiscectomy, lumbar decompression). The timing of surgery is essential. She also requires input from the neuro-urologist and physiotherapists.

Potential debates for discussion

Role of spinal fixation in cases of back pain without spondylolisthesis.

Role of discography in selecting patients for spinal fixation with 'discogenic' back pain.

Role and importance of urodynamic studies in identifying incomplete recovery from cauda equina syndrome.

Case 7: Pain pathways

A 43-year-old man underwent an elective craniotomy to debulk an underlying space-occupying lesion (SOL) 6 hours ago. He reports moderate headaches and sharp pain around the incision site.

What is pain and what are its mechanisms of transmission?

Pain is a physiological response to noxious stimuli (e.g. thermal, mechanical, chemical or trauma) that are damaging to the underlying tissues. Mechanisms of pain transmission are classified below.

- **Transduction** – the mechanism by which receptors are activated. Noxious stimulus is converted into electrochemical stimulus, which in turn is converted into an electrochemical impulse.

- **Transmission** – the mechanism by which an electrochemical impulse travels in the dorsal horn of the spinal cord to the thalamus and cortex.
- **Modulation** – the mechanism by which the pain impulse is dampened or amplified; occurs primarily in the dorsal horn of the spinal cord.
- **Perception** – refers to the subjective experience of pain that results from the interaction of transduction, transmission, modulation and the psychological aspects of the individual.

There are two main components of the spinothalamic tract (Figure 6.4).

1. The lateral spinothalamic tract transmits pain and temperature.
2. The anterior spinothalamic tract (or ventral spinothalamic tract) transmits crude touch and pressure.

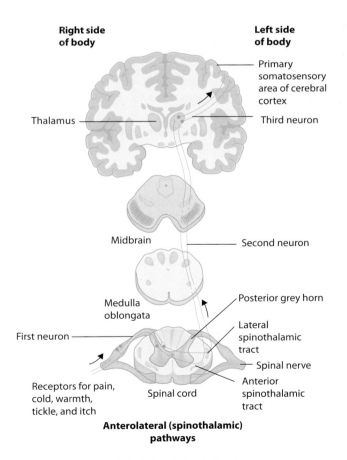

Figure 6.4 Spinothalamic tract.

The International Association for the Study of Pain (IASP) defines the following key pain terms:

Pain	An unpleasant sensory and emotional experience associated with actual or potential tissue damage, or described in terms of such damage.
Allodynia	Pain due to a stimulus that does not normally provoke pain.
Analgesia	Absence of pain in response to stimulation which would normally be painful.
Anesthesia dolorosa	Pain in an area or region that is anaesthetic.
Causalgia	A syndrome of sustained burning pain, allodynia, and hyperpathia after a traumatic nerve lesion, often combined with vasomotor and sudomotor dysfunction and later trophic changes.
Dysesthesia	An unpleasant abnormal sensation, whether spontaneous or evoked.
Hyperalgesia	Increased pain from a stimulus that normally provokes pain.
Hyperesthesia	Increased sensitivity to stimulation, excluding the special senses.
Hyperpathia	A painful syndrome characterized by an abnormally painful reaction to a stimulus, especially a repetitive stimulus, as well as an increased threshold.
Hypoalgesia	Diminished pain in response to a normally painful stimulus.
Hypoesthesia	Decreased sensitivity to stimulation, excluding the special senses.
Neuralgia	Pain in the distribution of a nerve or nerves.
Neuritis	Inflammation of a nerve or nerves.
Neuropathic pain	Pain caused by a lesion or disease of the somatosensory nervous system.
Neuropathy	A disturbance of function or pathological change in a nerve. (One nerve: mononeuropathy; several nerves: mononeuropathy multiplex; diffuse and bilateral: polyneuropathy.)
Nociception	The neural process of encoding noxious stimuli.
Nociceptive neuron	A central or peripheral neuron of the somatosensory nervous system that is capable of encoding noxious stimuli.
Nociceptive pain	Pain that arises from actual or threatened damage to non-neural tissue and is due to the activation of nociceptors.
Nociceptive stimulus	An actually or potentially tissue-damaging event transduced and encoded by nociceptors.
Nociceptor	A high-threshold sensory receptor of the peripheral somatosensory nervous system that is capable of transducing and encoding noxious stimuli.
Noxious stimulus	A stimulus that is damaging or threatens damage to normal tissues.
Pain threshold	The minimum intensity of a stimulus that is perceived as painful.
Pain tolerance level	The maximum intensity of a pain-producing stimulus that a subject is willing to accept in a given situation.
Paresthesia	An abnormal sensation, whether spontaneous or evoked.
Sensitization	Increased responsiveness of nociceptive neurons to their normal input, and/or recruitment of a response to normally subthreshold inputs.
Central sensitization	Increased responsiveness of nociceptive neurons in the central nervous system to their normal or subthreshold afferent input.
Peripheral sensitization	Increased responsiveness and reduced threshold of nociceptive neurons in the periphery to the stimulation of their receptive fields.

What is the 'gate control' theory?

In 1965, the gate control theory was described by Melzack and Wall. The theory explains that perception of physical pain is not a direct result of activation of nociceptors, but is rather modulated by interaction between different neurons, both pain-transmitting and non-pain-transmitting, in the substantia gelatinosa of the spinal cord. A gate control system modulates sensory input from the skin before it evokes pain perception and response.

- Aδ fibres are fast and myelinated (transmission occurs in 0.1 second, travels 6–30 m/s); they transmit pain as sharp and electric in nature.
- C fibres are slow and unmyelinated (transmission occurs after 1 second but increases over additional seconds to minutes, travels 0.05–2 m/s) and transmit pain as burning, aching or throbbing in nature.
- Aβ fibres are large-diameter fibres that are non-nociceptive (e.g. do not transmit pain stimuli) and inhibit the effects of Aδ and C fibres.

Large myelinated fibres have negative dorsal root potentials, and smaller C fibres have positive potentials. Stimulation of the larger fibres prevents transmission of pain impulses in the smaller fibres by maintaining a negative potential in the dorsal horn.

Potential debates for discussion

Utility of intrathecal morphine pumps.
Current indications and techniques of cordotomy.
Efficacy of occipital nerves stimulation.

Summary		
Allodynia	Lowered threshold	Stimulus and response mode differ.
Hyperalgesia	Increased response	Stimulus and response mode are similar.
Hyperpathia	Raised threshold: increased response	Stimulus and response mode may be the same or different.
Hypoalgesia	Raised threshold: lowered response	Stimulus and response mode are similar.

Case 8: Neuropharmacology

Case A

A 31-year-old man presents to the trauma centre after sustaining a gunshot wound to the head. The patient is immediately intubated, ventilated and sedated. On examination, his GCS was 3 with equal and reactive pupils. His CT scan demonstrates sulci effacement, diffuse subarachnoid blood, and a bullet fragment in the left parietal lobe. His EEG shows seizure activity. After 1 hour, his ICP readings continue to rise up to 40 cm H_2O.

Describe the pharmacology of the following medications, which are used to medically address his increased ICP and control seizures.

Mannitol

Mode of action
  An osmotic diuretic that results in an immediate plasma expansion. It reduces blood viscosity and haematocrit, which in turn increases CBF and O2 delivery, therefore improving the overall blood rheology.
  Causes an increase in the intravascular volume by drawing water from the cerebral parenchyma.
  A free-radical scavenger.
  Also supports the microcirculation.

Complications
  Opens the endothelial cells in the BBB, which can potentially aggravate vasogenic oedema.
  Hypertension.
  Hyperosmolar state leading to renal failure (e.g. acute tubular necrosis).
  Electrolyte derangement (e.g. hypernatraemia).

Phenytoin

Mode of action.
  Phenytoin blocks sustained high-frequency repetitive firing of action potentials. This is accomplished by reducing the amplitude of sodium-dependent action potentials through enhancing steady-state inactivation. Sodium channels exist in three main conformations (resting, open or inactive states). Phenytoin binds preferentially to the inactive form and blocks sodium channel.

Pharmacokinetics.
  Mixed-order kinetics at therapeutic concentrations.
  First-order kinetics at low levels.
  Zero-order kinetics at high levels.

Complications.
  - Allergy (fever, rash, polyarthritis).
  - Carcinongenesis.
  - Cerebellar dysfunction and degeneration (e.g. nystagmus, ataxia).
  - Cognitive dysfunction.
  - Coarse facial features.
  - Dermatological disorders (hypertrichosis and hirsutism).
  - Diplopia.
  - Gingival hypertrophy.
  - Haematological disorders (low folate levels, megaloblastic anaemia).
  - Hepatic granulomas.
  - Hypersensitivity.
  - Teratogenicity.
  - Systemic lupus erythematosus (SLE)-like syndrome.
  - Stevens–Johnson syndrome.
  - Stupor.
  - Peripheral neuropathy.

Signs of toxicity (use the mnemonic: SCAND):
  Slurred speech.
  Confusion – CNS depression.
  Asterixis.
  Nystagmus.
  Diplopia.

Carbamazepine

Mode of action.
  Carbamazepine stabilizes the inactive state of voltage-gated sodium channels and potentiates gamma-aminobutyric acid (GABA) receptors.

Pharmacokinetics.

Carbamazepine is relatively slowly but well absorbed after oral administration. Its plasma half-life is 20–55 hours when given as single dose, but it is a strong inducer of hepatic enzymes, and the plasma half-life shortens to ~15 hours when it is given repeatedly.

Complications.

- Drowsiness and gastrointestinal upset.
- Headache and migraines, motor coordination impairment.
- SIADH.
- Relative leukopenia.
- Haematological toxicity (agranulocytosis, aplastic anaemia).
- Hepatitis.
- Stevens–Johnson syndrome.
- Transient diplopia.
- Ataxia.

Case B

A 76-year-old man presents with tremor, rigidity, bradykinesia and recurrent falls

Select a medication used to treat Parkinson's disease and explain the pharmacology.

Sinemet

Sinemet (carbidopa-levodopa) is used to treat Parkinson's disease. **Carbidopa,** an inhibitor of aromatic amino acid decarboxylation, blocks the metabolism of levodopa in the liver, decreasing nausea and increasing the amount of levodopa that reaches the brain. **Levodopa,** an aromatic amino acid, is rapidly converted into dopamine by the enzyme dopa decarboxylase (DDC), which is present in the central and peripheral nervous systems. The majority of levodopa is metabolized before it reaches the brain. Levodopa is most effective in treating bradykinesia and rigidity, less effective in reducing tremor and improving gait imbalance. Side effects include abnormal muscle movement, chorea, confusion, depression, difficulty sleeping, dry mouth, dizzy spells, hallucinations, loss of appetite, nausea, sleepiness, vomiting and weakness.

What is the surgical treatment for Parkinson's disease?

Tissue transplantation (research phase)

Tissue transplantation involves the implantation of fetal dopaminergic brain cells into Parkinson's disease patients. Other options include using the patient's own adrenal medulla.

Pallidotomy

Pallidotomy directly destroys a portion of the internal segment of the globus pallidus (GPi), interrupting pallidofungal pathways or diminishing inputs to the medial pallidum (including the subthalamic nucleus).

Electrical stimulation

Electrical stimulation consists of deep brain stimulation (DBS) to the GPi and subthalamic nucleus (STN). Patients are considered for DBS if they have been refractory to medical treatment and their main symptoms are rigidity or bradykinesia. If tremor is also present, consider the ventralis intermedius (VIM) target.

Case C

A 59-year-old woman presents with a 3-week history of deterioration in her speech and left-sided weakness. Her MRI scan demonstrates a large enhancing frontal space-occupying lesion with significant oedema. She is started on dexamethasone. She undergoes a craniotomy to debulk her SOL. Formal histology confirms the diagnosis of a glioblastoma multiforme (GBM).

Describe the pharmacology of the following medications, which are used to medically address her cerebral oedema:

Dexamethasone

Mode of action.

Dexamethasone is a potent synthetic member of the glucocorticoid class of steroid drugs that has anti-inflammatory and immunosuppressant effects. It is 25 times more potent than cortisol in its glucocorticoid effect, while having minimal mineralocorticoid effect. Glucocorticoids enter cells through passive diffusion and form a complex with a receptor protein. This complex then undergoes an irreversible activation and enters the cell nucleus, where it binds to DNA, leading to biological effects induced by these hormones, including increased hepatic gluconeogenesis, increased lipolysis, muscle catabolism, and inhibition of peripheral glucose uptake in muscle and adipose tissue. In addition, dexamethasone increases angiopoietin-1 and decreases vascular endothelial growth factor (VEGF) in the endothelial cell.

Pharmokinetics.

Dexamethasone is metabolized by the liver. Its half-life is 1.8 to 3.5 hours.

Function.

- Reduce peritumoural and vasogenic brain oedema.
- Reduce increased intracranial pressure.
- Decrease frequency of plateau waves.
- Decrease cerebral spinal fluid production.
- Decrease tumour cerebral blood.

Complications.

- Gastrointestinal: gastritis and steroid ulceration, pancreatitis, intestinal perforation, elevated liver enzymes, fatty liver degeneration, hiccups.
- Cardiovascular and renal: hypertension, sodium and salt retention and hypokalemic acidosis.
- Central nervous system: progressive multifocal leukoencephalopathy (PML), mental agitation, epidural lipomatosis, pseudotumour cerebri.
- Endocrine: weight gain, hyperlipidaemia, Cushing's syndrome, glucose intolerance and diabetes mellitus.
- Ophthalmological: posterior subcapsular cataracts, glaucoma.
- Musculoskeletal: avascular necrosis, osteoporosis, muscle wasting.
- Haematological: hypercoagulopathy, demargination of white blood cells – increasing the white blood cell count, immunosuppressant action (pre-disposition to bacterial, viral, and fungal infections).
- Psychiatric disturbances: depression, personality changes, irritability, euphoria, or mania and mood swings.
- Dermatological: acne, allergic dermatitis, dry scaly skin, ecchymoses, petechiae, erythema, impaired wound healing, increased sweating, rash, striae, suppression of reactions to skin tests, thin fragile skin, thinning scalp hair, urticaria.

Potential debates for discussion

Role of steroids in spinal cord injuries.
Speed of action of steroids in tumoural brain oedema.
Role of steroids in non-tumoural brain oedema.

Interstitial chemotherapy with biodegradable BCNU (Gliadel) wafers

Mode of action.

The Gliadel wafer is a biodegradable slow-release drug-impregnated wafer containing carmustine or bis-chloroethylnitrosourea (BCNU). It is a mustard gas–related β-chloro-nitrosourea compound used as an alkylating agent in chemotherapy. Its cytostatic properties are secondary to its inhibitory effects at multiple levels, such as DNA, RNA and protein synthesis.

Pharmacokinetics.

After both oral and intravenous administration, BCNU has a very short life, with the parent drug not being detectable after 5 minutes, and its active metabolites detected in urine up to 72 hours after the initial dose. Both the parent drug and its metabolites rapidly enter the CSF. BCNU penetration inside the brain tissue is just for a very short distance (2 mm from the ependymal surface).

Complications.
- Postcraniotomy infection.
- Cerebral oedema.
- Pericavity necrosis.

Case 9: Informed consent

A 63-year-old man, who is unconscious, requires an emergency craniotomy to evacuate an extradural haematoma. A 7-year-old boy requires a revision of his ventriculoperitoneal (VP) shunt.

Who provides consent in these situations?

The 63-year-old is unconscious and requires an emergency operation. In the case of an unconscious patient, the next of kin should be notified. If no next of kin is available, it is best to obtain a colleague's agreement with the surgical procedure proposed and document this in the medical notes. The law recognizes that it is in the patient's best interest to go ahead with such an emergency treatment. In the case of the 7-year-old boy who requires a revision of his VP shunt, children under the age of 16 are legally unable to give consent, and the parent or guardian should provide consent on their behalf. The procedure and its potential benefits and risks should be explained to the child, parent or guardian.

What are the principles of consent?

- Informed consent means that the procedure is carefully explained to the patient in a balanced and unemotional way, stating the benefits and the significant risks associated with the procedure. Alternative treatments must also be explained.
- The patient has a legal right to withhold consent if of sound mind.

1. **Informed consent** – the patient has adequate information to make a decision.
   - Explain why you think a proposed treatment is necessary.
   - Explain the benefits and risks of the proposed treatment.
   - Explain what might happen if this treatment is not carried out.
   - Explain what other forms of treatment are available with their risks and benefits.

2. **Voluntary decision** – the patient has made the decision.
3. **Ability** – the patient has the ability to weigh the benefits and risks of surgery and make an informed decision.

What about children over the age of 16?

Once children reach the age of 16, they are presumed by the law to be competent. They are able to give consent for themselves for their own medical and surgical treatment along with any associated procedures, including investigations or anaesthesia. However, it is best practice to encourage competent children to involve their families in decision-making.

What is competency?

The patient comprehends, retains and weighs the information in order to make an informed decision regarding treatment.

What happens if a child aged 16 or 17 is not competent?

If a child is aged 16 or 17 and not competent to make an informed decision, then a person with parental responsibility can make the decision for him or her. However, the child should still be involved as much as possible in the process.

What happen when a child reaches the age of 18?

Once children reach the age of 18, no one else can make the decisions on their behalf. If an 18 year-old is not competent to make his or her own decisions, clinicians can provide treatment and care that is in the patient's 'best interest'.

What happens to a child under the age of 16?

Children younger than 16 are not automatically presumed to be legally competent to make decisions about their healthcare. However, the courts have stated that children under the age of 16 will be competent to give valid consent to a particular intervention if they have 'sufficient understanding and intelligence to enable him or her to understand fully what is proposed', known as 'Gillick competence'. As with older children, you must respect requests from a competent patient under the age of 16 by keeping his or her treatment confidential.

Should the consent form be signed?

Legally, it makes no difference whether the patient signs a form to indicate consent or whether they give consent orally or even non-verbally (e.g. holding out an arm for their blood pressure to be taken). A consent form is only a record, not proof that genuine consent has been given. It is best practice to seek written consent and to document this in the patient's medical notes.

When is it lawful to provide treatment based on the child's best interests?

- Emergency – no one with parental responsibility is available.

- Emergency – available parents not capable of providing informed consent (e.g. under influence of alcohol).

Potential debates for discussion

Blood transfusion in paediatric cases involving Jehovah's Witness families.

Case 10: Management of common neurosurgical conditions

Case A

An 83-year-old woman reports right-sided facial pain in the V1 and V2 distribution. She has been diagnosed with trigeminal neuralgia.

What are the management options of this condition?

Trigeminal neuralgia can be managed by medical and surgical treatment.

- Medical treatment: carbamazepine, gabapentin.
- Surgical treatment.
  - Peripheral nerve ablation or neurectomy.
  - Percutaneous trigeminal rhizotomy.
    - Chemical: glycerol injection into Meckel's cave.
    - Electrical: radiofrequency thermocoagulation.
    - Mechanical: balloon compression.
  - Microvascular decompression (MVD).
- Stereotactic radiosurgery.

The following factors will help in determining which treatment option is ideal for the patient:

- Age.
- Comorbidities.
- Failure of medical management.
- Patient's choice.

Potential debates for discussion

Efficacy, limitations and targets for stereotactic radiosurgery (STRS) in trigeminal neuralgia.

Case B

A 33-year-old woman reports headaches, visual deterioration and amenorrhea. She has been diagnosed with Cushing's disease (Figure 6.5).

What investigations should be performed for this condition?

The diagnosis of Cushing's disease should be confirmed. Obtain a detailed history and examine the cardiorespiratory and neurological systems. Collaboration with an endocrinologist is recommended. Further investigations include general and specific investigations.

General tests: full blood count, urea and electrolytes, urine dipstick (assess for glucose: diabetes), chest radiography and ECG.

Specific tests.

- Pituitary function test (prolactin, 8 a.m. cortisol, follicle-stimulating hormone [FSH], luteinizing hormone [LH], T4, thyroid-stimulating hormone [TSH], insulin-like growth factor-1 [IGF-1], fasting glucose).
- 24-hour of urine-free cortisol (suggestive of hypercortisolaemia if >3× normal).
- Overnight low-dose dexamethasone suppression test (to establish a primary or secondary cause).
- Adrenocorticotrophic hormone (ACTH) levels.
- Visual field assessment.
- Brain MRI scan.
- Further assessment: Synacten test (ACTH stimulation test) assesses the functioning of the adrenal gland stress response by measuring the adrenal response to ACTH. ACTH is a hormone produced in the anterior pituitary gland that stimulates the adrenal glands to release cortisol, dehydroepiandrosterone (DHEAS) and aldosterone. It is a useful investigation in cases of suspected reduced pituitary ACTH production reserve. It is used to diagnose or exclude primary and secondary adrenalin sufficiency, Addison's disease and related conditions. In addition to quantifying adrenal insufficiency, the test can distinguish whether the cause is adrenal (low cortisol and aldosterone production) or pituitary (low ACTH production).

- A synthetic analogue of ACTH, cosyntropin 0.25 mg, is administered by the intravenous or the intramuscular route.
- Cortisol levels are drawn before the dose is administered and again 30 minutes after administration.
- If the increase in cortisol is less than 6 mcg/dL, the hypothalamic-pituitary axis is still suppressed and the patient still requires supplementation for another 4 weeks. If the increase is greater than 6 mcg/dL, the patient no longer requires steroid therapy because adrenal function has returned to normal.
- Petrosal sampling procedure: in cases of diagnostic dilemma, you can confirm the source of ACTH and help predict the lateralization of Cushing's disease.

Post-operative morning cortisol levels are typically measured 72 hours after surgery. In the post-operative period, morning cortisol levels are typically low because normal ACTH-producing cells in the pituitary have been suppressed by elevated serum cortisol levels. Therefore, the removal of the ACTH-secreting tumour leaves no source of ACTH, the adrenal glands are no longer stimulated and cortisol levels drop. It is important to note that up to 30% of patients with long-term cure of Cushing's disease do not have a history of undetectable 72-hour post-operative serum cortisol levels. Therefore, if 72-hour post-operative cortisol levels are not below 5 μg/dL, further investigations are warranted to confirm cure.

What are the management options of this condition?

The treatment choice for Cushing's disease is transsphenoidal surgery performed by designated pituitary neurosurgeons. In cases where surgery is not possible or has failed, patients can be treated with medical therapy (ketoconazole), radiation or adrenalectomy.

Potential debates for discussion

Problems with total hypophysectomy (for the treatment of Cushing's disease) in young patients.
Role of radiotherapy in Nelson's syndrome.

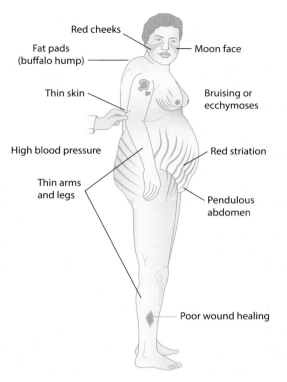

Figure 6.5 Signs of cushing's syndrome.

Case C

A 47-year-old man reports headaches, fatigue, and joint pain. His past medical history includes hypertension and carpal tunnel syndrome. He has been diagnosed with acromegaly.

What investigations should be performed for this condition?

The diagnosis of acromegaly should be confirmed. Obtain a detailed history and examine the cardiorespiratory and neurological systems. Collaboration with an endocrinologist is recommended. Further investigations include general and specific investigations.

General tests.
- Full blood count, urea and electrolytes, urine dipstick (assess for glucose: diabetes), chest radiography and ECG.

Specific tests.
- Pituitary function test (prolactin, 8 a.m. cortisol, FSH, LH, T4, TSH, IGF-1, fasting glucose).
- Growth hormone (GH): in acromegaly GH >10 ng/mL.
- IGF-1 (somatomedin): in acromegaly IGF-1> 6.8 U/mL.
- Glucose suppression test (oral glucose tolerance test [GTT]) – give 75 mg of glucose to the patient and then measure the serum GH levels every 30 minutes for 2 h. Positive test for acromegaly >5 mcg/L.
- Visual field assessment.
- Brain MRI scan.
- Further assessment: colonoscopy (due to increased risk of colonic polyps).

What are the management options of this condition?

Acromegaly should be managed by transsphenoidal surgery. Surgery provides a more rapid reduction in GH levels and decompresses the neural structures. In cases where surgery is not possible or has failed, patients can be treated with medical therapy. Dopamine agonists (bromocriptine, pegvisomant or octreotide) should be used. Radiation is reserved for patients in whom medical treatment has failed and should not be considered as an initial treatment.

Potential debates for discussion

Role of octreotide as a pre-operative adjunct.
Criteria for 'cure'.
Use of fractionated radiotherapy vs. gamma knife radiosurgery for relapses of acromegaly following surgery.

Case D

A 29-year-old man presents with new onset of seizures coupled with headaches. He has been diagnosed with arteriovenous malformation (AVM).

What are the management options of this condition?

Management is based on the following:

- Age of the patient.
- Comorbidities.
- Associated aneurysms (on feeding vessels, draining veins or intra-nidal).
- Flow (high or low).
- History of previous haemorrhage.
- Size and compactness of the nidus.
- Patient's wishes.

AVMs are managed by the following: conservative, medical, endovascular and surgical treatment. Surgery is the treatment choice for low-grade AVMs. The Spetzler–Martin classification grades AVMs according to their degree of surgical difficulty and the risk of surgical morbidity and mortality. The Spetzler–Martin AVM grading system allocates points for various features of intracranial AVMs to provide an overall score between 1 and 5. Grade 6 is used to describe inoperable lesions.

Spetzler–Martin grading system

Size of nidus.
Small (<3 cm) = 1.
Medium (3-6 cm) = 2.
Large (> 6 cm) = 3.

Eloquence of adjacent brain.
Non-eloquent = 0.
Eloquent = 1.

Venous drainage.
Superficial only = 0.
Deep = 1.

Eloquence of adjacent brain

Eloquence of brain: sensorimotor, language, visual cortex, hypothalamus, thalamus, brain stem, cerebellar nuclei, or regions directly adjacent to these structures.

Non-eloquence of brain: frontal and temporal lobe, cerebellar hemispheres.

Low-grade AVM: Grade I, II, III
High-grade AVM: Grade IV, V
Inoperative lesions: Grade VI

Three-tier classification of cerebral AVMS with treatment paradigm (2011).

Class	Spetzler–Martin Grade	Management
A	I & II	Resection
B	III	Multimodality treatment
C	IV & V	No treatment

Potential debates for discussion

Results for epilepsy control after stereotactic radiosurgery (STRS) for AVMs.
Influence of combined endovascular embolization on obliteration rates after STRS for AVMs.

References

Spetzler M, Martin N. A proposed grading system for arteriovenous malformations. *J Neurosurg* 1986; 65: 476–483.

Spetzler RF, Ponce FA. A 3-tier classification of cerebral arteriovenous malformations. Clinical article. *J Neurosurg* 2011; 114(3): 842–849.

Case E

A 45-year-old woman presents with unilateral hearing loss and tinnitus. She has been diagnosed with vestibular schwannoma.

What are the management options of this condition?

Vestibular schwannomas are managed by the following: conservative, radiation and surgical treatment.

The two most popular management options have the following profile:

Microsurgery.
>97% chance of complete tumour removal.
95% of patients with small tumours retaining House-Brackmann Grade I or II facial function.
50% retaining useful hearing.

Radiosurgery.
90% of cases: vestibular schwannoma will stop growing.
98% of cases: no facial nerve palsy.
75% will retain useful hearing.

The major determinants of which treatment is adopted are the following:
- Tumour size.
- Age of the patient.
- Comorbidities.
- Hearing preservation.
- State of the hearing in the contralateral ear.
- Patient's wishes.

Potential debates for discussion

Hearing assessment.
Management of bilateral vestibular schwannomas in neurofibromatosis type II (NF-2) cases for tumour control and hearing preservation.

Reference

Rutherford SA, King AT. Vestibular schwannoma management: what is the "best" options? *Br J Neurosurg* 2005; 19(4): 309–316.

Case F

A 17-year-old boy presents with a 2-week history of progressive headaches associated with nausea and vomiting. His MRI scan demonstrates a homogeneous and hyperintense mass in the pineal region with associated hydrocephalus.

What are the management options of this condition?

Initial management of patients with pineal region tumours should be directed at treating hydrocephalus and establishing a diagnosis of the underlying pineal tumour. The treatment of the hydrocephalus depends on the patient's clinical state and subsequent definitive treatment plan. Options include close observation while awaiting surgery, ventriculoscopy or EVD, endoscopic third ventriculostomy, (ETV), or a VP shunt. A third ventriculostomy has the added advantage of potentially allowing for an open biopsy during the procedure by endoscopic guidance.

Preoperative evaluation should include the following:

- A high-resolution brain MRI scan with gadolinium.
- Measurement of serum and CSF markers.
- Cytology examination of CSF.
- Evaluation of pituitary function, if endocrine abnormalities are suspected.
- Visual field examination if suprasellar extension of the tumour is demonstrated on the MRI scan. The ultimate management goal should be to refine adjuvant therapy based on tumour pathology.

Serum and CSF tumour markers:

> Alpha-fetoprotein is commonly elevated in the following:
>> Yolk sac tumours.
>> Embryonal cell carcinoma.
>> Immature teratoma.

> Beta-human chorionic gonadotropin is commonly elevated in the following:
>> Choriocarcinoma.
>> Germinoma with syncytiotrophoblasts.
>> Embryonal cell carcinomas.

> Placental alkaline phosphatase is commonly elevated in the following:
>> Germinomas.
>> May be positive in all germ cell tumours (GCTs).

The common surgical approaches include infratentorial supracerebellar, occipital transtentorial and transcallosal interhemispheric. Radiotherapy is indicated for all patients with germinomas, malignant germ cell tumours, malignant or intermediate pineal cell tumours, anaplastic gliomas, or subtotal resection of pineocytoma or ependymomas. Chemotherapy (usually combined with radiotherapy) is used in germinoma, nongerminomatous GCTs, germinoma with syncytiotrophoblastic cells, and recurrent or metastatic germinoma or pineal cell tumours.

Potential debates for discussion

> Diagnosis and management of incidental pineal cysts.
> Role of tumour markers in precluding a tissue diagnosis.
> Likely diagnosis (statistically) and management in a patient with a pineal tumour and elevated ß-HCG levels.

Case G

A 55-year-old woman presents with a sudden onset of a severe headache coupled with vomiting and photophobia. Her CT scan demonstrates an extensive subarachnoid haemorrhage (SAH).

What are the management options of this condition?

The patient is treated with hypervolemia, hypertension and haemodilution. Nimodipine (60 mg PO every 4 hours for 21 days) should be commenced. If there is clinical and radiological evidence of hydrocephalus, an EVD should be inserted. Further investigations include computed tomography angiography (CTA), transcranial Doppler and a formal cerebral angiogram. Treatment can be conservative, medical, endovascular or surgical. In patients with a ruptured intracranial aneurysm, the outcome (survival free of disability at 1 year) is better with endovascular coiling compared to clipping.

	Endovascular (%)	Surgery (%)
Dependent or dead at 1 year	23.7	30.6
Relative and absolute risk reductions in dependency or death	22.6	6–9

What is the grading system for SAH?

Hunt and Hess grading.

Grade	Clinical condition
0	Unruptured
I	Asymptomatic or minimal headache, nuchal rigidity
II	Moderate to severe headache, nuchal rigidity, no neurological deficit other than cranial nerve palsy
III	Drowsiness, confusion, mild focal deficit
IV	Stupor, moderate to severe hemiparesis, possible early decerebrate rigidity and vegetative disturbances
V	Deep coma, decerebrate rigidity, moribund appearance

World Federation of Neurological Surgeons (WFNS) grading.

WFNS grades	GCS score	Motor deficit
I	15	Absent
II	14–13	Absent
III	14–13	Present
IV	12–7	Present or absent
V	6–3	Present or absent

References

Molyneux A, Kerr R, Stratton I et al. (International Subarachnoid Aneurysm Trial [ISAT] Collaborative Group). International Subarachnoid Aneurysm Trial (ISAT) of neurosurgical clipping versus endovascular coiling in 2143 patients with ruptured intracranial aneurysms: a randomised trial. *Lancet* 2002; 360: 1267–1274.

Case H

A 53-year-old woman presents with a 3-year history of headaches. She is a smoker and has a family history of cerebral aneurysms.

What is the natural history of unruptured aneurysms?

Risk of rupture depends on the following:

- Size: The most important predictor for future rupture.
  - <10 mm in diameter: 0.05%/year.
  - >10 mm in diameter: 1%/year.

A follow-up by the International Study of Unruptured Intracranial Aneurysms Investigators stated the 5-year cumulative rupture rate for patients with unruptured aneurysms.

Size of unruptured aneurysm	<7	7–12	13–24	>24 mm
Anterior circulation	0	2.6	14.5	40%
Posterior circulation	2.5	14.5	18.4	50%

- Site: posterior communicating artery (PCoA), vertebrobasilar and basilar termination unruptured aneurysms are more likely to rupture.
- Morphology: irregular and multi-lobular aneurysms are more likely to rupture.

What are the principles of screening? In the general population, is there a screening test for cerebral aneurysms?

Principles of screening are a test performed on asymptomatic individuals that allows for early detection, therapeutic intervention, and decreased mortality from the disease.

Wilson's criteria (World Health Organization guidelines)

- The condition should be an important health problem.
- The natural history of the condition should be understood.
- There should be a recognizable latent or early symptomatic stage.
- There should be a test that is easy to perform and interpret, acceptable, accurate, reliable, sensitive and specific.
- There should be an accepted treatment recognized for the disease.
- Treatment should be more effective if started early.
- There should be a policy on who should be treated.
- Diagnosis and treatment should be cost-effective.
- Case-finding should be a continuous process.

Screening of cerebral aneurysms is not established.

- The natural history is not known. We do not know how rapidly an aneurysm forms. It may be days, weeks or months. Therefore, even after a negative angiogram, there is no evidence that an aneurysm will not form.
- Screening technology is not sensitive enough to detect small aneurysms.
- Small aneurysms have a small rupture risk.
- Aneurysm treatment is not without risk.
- This has repercussions for applications for mortgage and life insurance.

Screening in patients with familiar intracranial aneurysms is controversial. Recently, evidence suggests that screening may be of benefit to female patients who have a positive family history (first-degree relative) who are in their fourth decade or older and have a history of smoking or hypertension. Magnetic resonance angiography (MRA) is the investigation of choice because it is less invasive and more cost effective compared to cerebral angiography.

Potential debates for discussion

Frequency of serial imaging in unruptured intracranial aneurysms managed conservatively.

References

Wiebers D, Whisnant J, Forbes G *et al.* (International Study of Unruptured Intracranial Aneurysms Investigators). Unruptured intracranial aneurysms – risk of rupture and risks of surgical intervention. *N Engl J Med* 1998; 339(24): 1725–1733.

Wiebers DO, Whisnant JP, Houston J et al. (International Study of Unruptured Intracranial Aneurysms Investigators.) Unruptured intracranial aneurysms: natural history, clinical outcome, and risks of surgical and endovascular treatment. *Lancet* 2003; 362: 103–110.

7

Landmark publications

We recommend that you be familiar with these landmark publications.

Functional

Benabid AL, Pollak P, Gao D, *et al*. Chronic electrical stimulation of the ventralis intermedius nucleus of the thalamus as a treatment of movement disorders. *J Neurosurg* 1996; 84(2): 203–214.

Benabid AL, Pollak P, Louveau A, *et al*. Combined (thalamotomy and stimulation) stereotactic surgery of the VIM thalamic nucleus for bilateral Parkinson disease. *Appl Neurophysiol* 1987; 50(1–6): 344–346.

Coubes P, Roubertie A, Vayssiere N, *et al*. Treatment of DYT1-generalised dystonia by stimulation of the internal globus pallidus. *Lancet* 2000; 355(9222): 2220–2221.

Leksell L. The stereotaxic method and radiosurgery of the brain. *Acta Chir Scand* 1951; 102(4): 316–319.

Limousin P, Pollak P, Benazzouz A, *et al*. Bilateral subthalamic nucleus stimulation for severe Parkinson's disease. *Mov Disord* 1995; 10(5): 672–674.

May A, Bahra A, Büchel C, *et al*. Hypothalamic activation in cluster headache attacks. *Lancet* 1998; 352(9124): 275–278.

Wiebe S, Blume WT, Girvin JP, *et al*. (Effectiveness and Efficiency of Surgery for Temporal Lobe Epilepsy Study Group). A randomized, controlled trial of surgery for temporal-lobe epilepsy. *N Engl J Med* 2001; 345(5): 311–318.

Hydrocephalus

Adams RD, Fisher CM, Hakim S, *et al*. Symptomatic occult hydrocephalus with "normal" cerebro-spinal-fluid pressure. A treatable syndrome. *N Engl J Med* 1965; 273: 117–126.

Brodbelt A, Stoodley M. CSF pathways: a review. *Br J Neurosurg* 2007; 21(5): 510–520.

Oncology

Daumas-Duport C, Scheithauer B, O'Fallon J, *et al*. Grading of astrocytomas. A simple and reproducible method. *Cancer* 1988; 62(10): 2152–2165.

Hegi ME, Diserens AC, Gorlia T, *et al*. MGMT gene silencing and benefit from temozolomide in glioblastoma. *N Engl J Med* 2005; 352(10): 997–1003.

Keles GE, Lamborn KR, Berger MS. Low-grade hemispheric gliomas in adults: a critical review of extent of resection as a factor influencing outcome. *J Neurosurg* 2001; 95(5): 735–745.

Lacroix M, Abi-Said D, Fourney DR, *et al*. A multivariate analysis of 416 patients with glioblastoma multiforme: prognosis, extent of resection, and survival. *J Neurosurg* 2001; 95(2): 190–198.

Lagerwaard FJ, Levendag PC, Nowak PJ, *et al*. Identification of prognostic factors in patients with brain metastases: a review of 1292 patients. *Int J Radiat Oncol Biol Phys* 1999; 43(4): 795–803.

Louis DN, Ohgaki H, Wiestler OD, *et al.* The 2007 WHO classification of tumours of the central nervous system. *Acta Neuropathol* 2007; 114(2): 97–109.

Patchell RA, Tibbs PA, Walsh JW, *et al.* A randomized trial of surgery in the treatment of single metastases to the brain. *N Engl J Med* 1990; 322(8): 494–500.

Simpson D. The recurrence of intracranial meningiomas after surgical treatment. *J Neurol Neurosurg Psychiatry* 1957; 20(1): 22–39.

Stummer W, Pichlmeier U, Meinel T, *et al.* (for the ALA-Glioma Study Group). Fluorescence-guided surgery with 5-aminolevulinic acid for resection of malignant glioma: a randomised controlled multicentre phase III trial. *Lancet Oncol* 2006; 7(5): 392–401.

Stupp R, Mason WP, Bent MJ, *et al.* Radiotherapy plus concomitant and adjuvant temozolomide for glioblastoma. *N Engl J Med* 2005; 352: 987–996.

Walker MD, Alexander E Jr, Hunt WE, *et al.* Evaluation of BCNU and/or radiotherapy in the treatment of anaplastic gliomas. A cooperative clinical trial. *J Neurosurg* 1978; 49(3): 333–343.

Walker MD, Green SB, Byar DP, *et al.* Randomized comparisons of radiotherapy and nitrosoureas for the treatment of malignant glioma after surgery. *N Engl J Med* 1980; 303(23): 1323–1329.

Yaşargil MG, Kadri PA, Yaşargil DC. Microsurgery for malignant gliomas. *J Neurooncol* 2004; 69(1–3): 67–81.

Yung WK, Albright RE, Olson J, *et al.* A phase II study of temozolomide vs. procarbazine in patients with glioblastoma multiforme at first relapse. *Br J Cancer* 2000; 83: 588–593.

Other

Collen JF, Jackson JL, Shorr AF *et al.* Prevention of venous thromboembolism in neurosurgery: a metaanalysis. *Chest* 2008; 134: 237–249.

Skull base

Barker FG, Jannetta PJ, Bissonette DJ. The long-term outcome of microvascular decompression for trigeminal neuralgia. *N Engl J Med* 1996; 334(17): 1077–1083.

Bills DC, Meyer FB, Laws ER Jr, *et al.* A retrospective analysis of pituitary apoplexy. *Neurosurgery* 1993; 33(4): 602–608; discussion 608–609.

Cappabianca P, Cavallo LM, de Divitiis E. Endoscopic endonasal transsphenoidal surgery. *Neurosurgery* 2004; 55(4): 933–940; discussion 940–941.

Hardy DG, Rhoton AL. Microsurgical relationships of the superior cerebellar artery and the trigeminal nerve. *J Neurosurg* 1978; 49(5): 669–678.

House JW, Brackmann DE. Facial nerve grading system. *Otolaryngol Head Neck Surg* 1985; 93(2): 146–147.

Jannetta PJ. Arterial compression of the trigeminal nerve at the pons in patients with trigeminal neuralgia. *J Neurosurg* 1967; 26(1): 159–162.

National Institutes of Health Consensus Development Conference. *Acoustic Neuroma: Consensus statement.* NIH Consens Dev Conf Consens Statement, Vol. 9. 1991.

Rhoton AL. The cerebellopontine angle and posterior fossa cranial nerves by the retrosigmoid approach. *Neurosurgery* 2000; 47(3 Suppl): S93–129.

Rhoton AL. Microsurgical anatomy of the brainstem surface facing an acoustic neuroma. *Surg Neurol* 1986; 25: 326–339.

Ross DA, Wilson CB. Results of transsphenoidal microsurgery for growth hormone-secreting pituitary adenoma in a series of 214 patients. *J Neurosurg* 1998; 68(6): 854–867.

Rutherford SA, King AT. Vestibular schwannoma management: what is the "best" option? *Br J Neurosurg* 2005; 19(4): 309–316.

Spine

Bracken MB, Shepard MJ, Collins WF, *et al.* A randomized, controlled trial of methylprednisolone or naloxone in the treatment of acute spinal-cord injury: Results of the Second National Acute Spinal Cord Injury Study. *N Engl J Med* 1990; 322(20): 1405–1411.

Legaye J, Duval-Beaupère G, Hecquet J, *et al.* Pelvic incidence: a fundamental pelvic parameter for three-dimensional regulation of spinal sagittal curves. *Eur Spine J* 1998; 7(2): 99–103.

Lenke LG, Betz RR, Harmes J, *et al.* Adolescent idiopathic scoliosis: a new classification to determine extent of spinal arthrodesis. *J Bone Joint Surg Am* 2001; 83(8): 1169–1181.

Patchell RA, Tibbs PA, Regine WF, *et al.* Direct decompressive surgical resection in the treatment of spinal cord compression caused by metastatic cancer: a randomised trial. *Lancet* 2005; 366(9486): 643–648.

Weinstein JN, Lurie JD, Tosteson TD, *et al.* Surgical versus nonsurgical therapy for lumbar spinal stenosis. *N Engl J Med* 2008; 358(8): 794–810.

Weinstein JN, Lurie JD, Tosteson TD, *et al.* Surgical versus nonsurgical treatment for lumbar degenerative spondylolisthesis. *N Engl J Med* 2007; 356: 2257–2270.

Weinstein JN, Tosteson TD, Lurie JD *et al.* Surgical vs nonoperative treatment for lumbar disk herniation: the Spine Patient Outcomes Research Trial (SPORT): a randomized trial. *JAMA* 2006; 296(20): 2441–2450.

Stroke

Aaslid R, Markwalder TM, Nornes H. Noninvasive transcranial Doppler ultrasound recording of flow velocity in basal cerebral arteries. *J Neurosurg* 1981; 57(6): 769–774.

Barnett HJ, Taylor DW, Eliasziw M, *et al.* Benefit of carotid endarterectomy in patients with symptomatic moderate or severe stenosis. North American Symptomatic Carotid Endarterectomy Trial Collaborators. *N Engl J Med* 1998; 339(20): 1415–1425.

European Carotid Surgery Trialists Collaboration Group. Randomised trial of endarterectomy for recently symptomatic carotid stenosis: final results of the MRC European Carotid Surgery Trial (ECST). *Lancet* 1998; 351(9113): 1379–1387.

Executive Committee for the Asymptomatic Carotid Atherosclerosis Study. Endarterectomy for asymptomatic carotid artery stenosis. *JAMA* 1995; 273(18): 1421–1428.

Ferguson GG, Eliasziw M, Barr HW, *et al.* The North American Symptomatic Carotid Endarterectomy Trial: surgical results in 1415 patients. *Stroke* 1999; 30(9): 1751–1758.

Kirollos RW, Tyagi AK, Ross SA, et al. Management of spontaneous cerebellar hematomas: a prospective treatment protocol. *Neurosurgery* 2001; 49(6): 1378–1386; discussion 1386–1387.

Mayberg MR, Wilson SE, Yatsu F, *et al.* Carotid endarterectomy and prevention of cerebral ischemia in symptomatic carotid stenosis. Veterans Affairs Cooperative Studies Program 309 Trialist Group. *JAMA* 1991; 266(23): 3289–3294.

Mendelow AD, Gregson BA, Fernandes HM, *et al.* (STICH investigators). Early surgery versus initial conservative treatment in patients with spontaneous supratentorial intracerebral haematomas in the International Surgical Trial in Intracerebral Haemorrhage (STICH): a randomised trial. *Lancet* 2005; 365(9457): 387–397.

North American Symptomatic Carotid Endarterectomy Trial Collaborators. Beneficial effect of carotid endarterectomy in symptomatic patients with high-grade carotid stenosis. *N Engl J Med* 1991; 325(7): 445–453.

Vahedi K, Hofmeijer J, Juettler E, *et al.* (DECIMAL, DESTINY, and HAMLET investigators). Early decompressive surgery in malignant infarction of the middle cerebral artery: a pooled analysis of three randomised controlled trials. *Lancet Neurol* 2007; 6(3): 215–222.

Trauma

Bouma GJ, Muizelaar JP, Bandoh K, *et al.* Blood pressure and intracranial pressure-volume dynamics in severe head injury: relationship with cerebral blood flow. *J Neurosurg* 1992; 77(1): 15–19.

Chesnut RM, Marshall LF, Klauber MR, *et al.* The role of secondary brain injury in determining outcome from severe head injury. *J Trauma* 1993; 34(2): 216–222.

Clifton GL, Miller ER, Choi SC, *et al.* Lack of effect of induction of hypothermia after acute brain injury. *N Engl J Med* 2001; 344(8): 556–563.

Cooper DJ, Rosenfeld JV, Murray L, *et al.* (The DECRA Trial Investigators and the Australian and New Zealand Intensive Care Society Clinical Trials Group). Decompressive craniectomy in diffuse traumatic brain injury. *N Engl J Med* 2011; 364(16): 1493–1502.

Edwards P, Arango M, Balica L, *et al.* (CRASH trial collaborators). Final results of MRC CRASH, a randomised placebo-controlled trial of intravenous corticosteroid in adults with head injury-outcomes at 6 months. *Lancet* 2005; 365(9475): 1957–1959.

Guerra WK, Gaab MR, Dietz H, *et al.* Surgical decompression for traumatic brain swelling: indications and results. *J Neurosurg* 1999; 90(2): 187–196.

Jennett B, Bond M. Assessment of outcome after severe brain damage. *Lancet* 1975; 1(7905): 480–484.

Marmarou A, Anderson RL, Ward JD. Impact of ICP instability and hypotension on outcome in patients with severe head trauma. *J Neurosurg* 1991; 75: S59–S66.

Maynard FM Jr, Bracken MB, Creasey G, *et al.* International Standards for Neurological and Functional Classification of Spinal Cord Injury. American Spinal Injury Association. *Spinal Cord* 1997; 35(5): 266–274.

Muizelaar JP, Marmarou A, Ward JD, *et al.* Adverse effects of prolonged hyperventilation in patients with severe head injury: a randomized clinical trial. *J Neurosurg* 1991; 75(5): 731–739.

Murray GD, Teasdale GM, Braakman R, *et al.* The European Brain Injury Consortium survey of head injuries. *Acta Neurochir* 1999; 141(3): 223–236.

Polin RS, Shaffrey ME, Bogaev CA, *et al.* Decompressive bifrontal craniectomy in the treatment of severe refractory post-traumatic cerebral edema. *Neurosurgery* 1997; 41(1): 84–92; discussion 92–94.

Roberts I, Yates D, Sandercock P, *et al.* Effect of intravenous corticosteroids on death within 14 days in 10 008 adults with clinically significant head injury (MRC CRASH trial): randomised placebo-controlled trial. *Lancet* 2004; 364(9442): 1321–1328.

Rosner MJ, Rosner SD, Johnson AH. Cerebral perfusion pressure: management protocol and clinical results. *J Neurosurg* 1995; 83(6): 949–962.

SAFE Study Investigators; Australian and New Zealand Intensive Care Society Clinical Trials Group, Australian Red Cross Blood Service, George Institute for International Health. Saline or albumin for fluid resuscitation in patients with traumatic brain injury. *N Engl J Med* 2007; 357(9): 874–884.

Santarius T, Kirkpatrick PJ, Ganesan D, *et al.* Use of drains versus no drains after burr-hole evacuation of chronic subdural haematoma: a randomised controlled trial. *Lancet* 2009; 374(9695): 1067–1073.

Teasdale G, Jennett B. Assessment of coma and impaired consciousness. A practical scale. *Lancet* 1974; 2(7872): 81–84.

Wilberger JE Jr, Harris M, Diamond DL. Acute subdural hematoma: morbidity, mortality, and operative timing. *J Neurosurg* 1991; 74(2): 212–218.

Vascular

Allen GS, Ahn HS, Preziosi TJ, *et al.* Cerebral arterial spasm – a controlled trial of nimodipine in patients with subarachnoid hemorrhage. *N Engl J Med* 1983; 308(11): 619–624.

Awad IA, Carter LP, Spetzler RF, *et al.* Clinical vasospasm after subarachnoid hemorrhage: response to hypervolemic hemodilution and arterial hypertension. *Stroke* 1987; 18(2): 365–372.

Barrow DL, Spector RH, Braun IF, *et al.* Classification and treatment of spontaneous carotid-cavernous fistulas. *J Neurosurg* 1985; 62: 248–256.

Diringer MN, Bleck, TP, Hemphill JC, *et al.* Critical care management of patients following aneurysmal subarachnoid hemorrhage: recommendations from the Neurocritical Care Society's Multidisciplinary Consensus Conference. *Neurocrit Care* 2011; 15: 211–240.

Fisher CM, Kistler JP, Davis JM. Relation of cerebral vasospasm to subarachnoid hemorrhage visualized by computerized tomographic scanning. *Neurosurgery* 1980; 6(1): 1–9.

Gobin YP, Laurent A, Merienne L, *et al.* Treatment of brain arteriovenous malformations by embolization and radiosurgery. *J Neurosurg* 1996; 85(1): 19–28.

Guglielmi G, Viñuela F, Dion, J, *et al.* Electrothrombosis of saccular aneurysms via endovascular approach. Part 2: Preliminary clinical experience. *J Neurosurg* 1991; 75(1): 8–14.

Juvela S, Porras M, Heiskanen O. Natural history of unruptured intracranial aneurysms: a long-term follow-up study. *J Neurosurg* 1993; 79(2): 174–182.

Kassell NF, Torner JC, Haley EC, *et al*. The International Cooperative Study on the Timing of Aneurysm Surgery. Part 1: Overall management results. *J Neurosurg.* 1990; 73(1): 18–36.

Kassell NF, Torner JC, Jane JA. The International Cooperative Study on the Timing of Aneurysm Surgery. Part 2: Surgical results. *J Neurosurg* 2010; 112(2): 37–47.

Mast H, Young WL, Koennecke HC, *et al*. Risk of spontaneous haemorrhage after diagnosis of cerebral arteriovenous malformation. *Lancet* 1997; 350(9084): 1065–1068.

McDougall CG, Spetzler RF, Zabramski JM, *et al*. The Barrow Ruptured Aneurysm Trial. *J Neurosurg* 2012; 116(1): 135–144.

Molyneux A, Kerr R, Stratton I, *et al*. (International Subarachnoid Aneurysm Trial (ISAT) Collaborative Group). International Subarachnoid Aneurysm Trial (ISAT) of neurosurgical clipping versus endovascular coiling in 2143 patients with ruptured intracranial aneurysms: a randomised trial. *Lancet* 2002; 360(9342): 1267–1274.

Pickard JD, Murray GD, Illingworth R, *et al*. Effect of oral nimodipine on cerebral infarction and outcome after subarachnoid haemorrhage: British aneurysm nimodipine trial. *BMJ* 1989; 298(6674): 636–642.

Solenski NJ, Haley EC Jr, Kassell NF, *et al*. Medical complications of aneurysmal subarachnoid hemorrhage: a report of the Multicenter, Cooperative Aneurysm Study. Participants of the Multicenter Cooperative Aneurysm Study. *Crit Care Med* 1995; 23(6): 1007–1017.

Spetzler RF, Martin NA. A proposed grading system for arteriovenous malformations. *J Neurosurg* 1986; 65(4): 476–483.

Spetzler RF, Ponce FA. A 3-tier classification of cerebral arteriovenous malformations. *J Neurosurg* 2011; 114(3): 842–849.

Stapf C. The rationale behind "A Randomized Trial of Unruptured Brain AVMs" (ARUBA). *Acta Neurochir Suppl* 2010; 107: 83–85.

Wiebers D, Whisnant J, Forbes G, *et al* (International Study Unruptured Intracranial Aneurysms Investigators). Unruptured intracranial aneurysms – risk of rupture and risks of surgical intervention. *N Engl J Med* 1998; 339(24): 1725–1733.

Wiebers DO, Whisnant JP, Huston J, *et al*. (International Study of Unruptured Intracranial Aneurysms Investigators). Unruptured intracranial aneurysms: natural history, clinical outcome, and risks of surgical and endovascular treatment. *Lancet* 2003; 362(9378): 103–110.

8

Key terms

Arachnoid cyst – cerebrospinal fluid covered by arachnoid cells and collagen. It is benign and occurs in the cerebrospinal axis in relation to the arachnoid membrane. It does not communicate with the ventricular system.

Atherosis – a continuous stream of slow writhing movements, typically of the hands and feet, often caused by damage to the corpus striatum.

Chiari malformation – a condition characterized by a downward displacement of the cerebellar tonsils and the medulla through the foramen magnum sometimes causing obstructive hydrocephalus as a result of obstruction of cerebral spinal fluid (CSF) outflow.

- Chiari Type 0 is the absence of the tonsils below the foramen magnum. It includes the presence of symptoms and a syrinx in the spinal cord. Controversial.
- Chiari Type 1, the most common type, is due to impaired CSF circulation through the foramen magnum. Commonly, the cerebral tonsillar herniation is >5 mm below the foramen magnum. In 30–70 per cent, there is an associated syringomyelia.
- Chiari Type 2, Arnold–Chiari malformation, results in caudally dislocated cervicomedullary junction, pons, fourth ventricle and medulla. The cerebellar tonsils are located at or below the foramen magnum. Usually associated with a myelomeningocele.
- Chiari Type 3, most severe form, results in the displacement of the posterior fossa structures, with cerebellum herniation through the foramen magnum into cervical canal. It is often associated with a high cervical or suboccipital encephalomeningocele.
- Chiari Type 4 is cerebellar hypoplasia without cerebellar herniation.

Chiari malformation Type 1 and 2

	Type 1	Type 2	
Age of presentation	Young adult	Child	
Usual presentation	Neck pain/ headaches	Hydrocephalus/respiratory distress	
Caudal dislocation of medulla	–	+	
Caudal dislocation into cervical canal	Tonsils	Inferior vermis, medulla, 4th ventricle	
Hydrocephalus	–	+	
Medullary 'kink'	–	+ (50%)	
Course of upper cranial nerves	Normal	Cephalad	

Chorea – an involuntary movement disorder characterized by brief, irregular contractions that are not repetitive or rhythmic, but appear to flow from one muscle to the next.

Colloid cyst – a benign, epithelium-lined cyst believed to originate from the anterior part of the third ventricle. The cysts are believed to derive from either primitive neuroepithelium of the tela choroidea or from the endoderm. Because of its location, it can cause obstructive hydrocephalus and increased intracranial pressure.

Craniopharyngioma – a benign, epithelium-lined cyst believed to originate from the anterior margin of the sella turcica. It has a benign histology and malignant behaviour.

- Embryogenetic theory suggests that the adamantinomatous type ('adamantinoma') arises from epithelial remnants of the involuted Rathke's pouch or the craniopharyngeal duct.
- Metaplastic theory suggests that the squamous papillary type results due to the metaplasia of residual squamous epithelium that arises from squamous cell nests normally found at the junction of the pituitary stalk and pars distalis.

Dermoid and epidermoid cysts – not true neoplasms, but are inclusion cysts composed of ectodermal elements as a result of a developmental abnormality. Centrally, they contain desquamated epithelial keratin and lipid material. The external surface is smooth, lobulated and pearly in appearance. They are lined with stratified squamous epithelium and contain an outer connective tissue capsule. Cyst characteristics and location distinguish them.

- Dermoid tumours include other dermal elements (hair, teeth, follicles, sebaceous glands) and they are located near the midline. They are associated with other congenital anomalies in up to 50 per cent of cases.
- Epidermoids are located laterally. They tend to be isolated lesions.

Dural arteriovenous fistula – an abnormal direct connection (fistula) between a meningeal artery and a meningeal vein or dural venous sinus. The Borden classification of dural arteriovenous malformations or fistulas is based on the venous drainage.

- Type I: dural arterial supply drains anterograde into venous sinus.
- Type II: dural arterial supply drains into venous sinus. High pressure in sinus results in both anterograde drainage and retrograde drainage via subarachnoid veins.
- Type III: dural arterial supply drains retrograde into subarachnoid veins.

Ependymoma – a glial tumour that arises from ependymal cells lining the cerebral ventricles and the central canal of the spinal cord. In the paediatric population, it tends to be located intracranially (fourth ventricle). In the adult population, it tends to be located in the spine.

Haemangioblastoma – a benign, highly vascular tumour that can occur in the brain and spine. It is composed of endothelial cells, pericytes and stromal cells. Most haemangioblastomas are single lesions. They can be associated with von Hippel–Lindau disease (VHL; see below).

Diagnostic criteria of von Hippel-Lindau disease (VHL)

Patients without a family history of VHL
- Two or more CNS haemangioblastomas
- One CNS haemangioblastoma and a visceral tumour (excluding epididymal or renal cysts)

Patients with a family history of VHL
- One CNS haemangioblastoma

    or
- Phaeochromocytoma

    or
- Clear cell renal carcinoma

Hemiballismus – a unilateral wild, large-amplitude flinging involuntary movement of the proximal part of the limbs, which results in postural imbalance. It is caused by a decrease in activity of the subthalamic nucleus of the basal ganglia.

Hydromyelia – a fluid collection within the spinal cord lined by ependymal cells.

Idiopathic intracranial hypertension – a condition characterized by increased intracranial pressure without evidence of intracranial mass, infection, hydrocephalus or hypertensive encephalopathy.

Medulloblastoma – one of the family of primitive neuroectodermal tumours (PNETs). This tumour is the most common paediatric brain malignancy and the most common PNET. It usually arises in the roof of the fourth ventricle, which can lead to hydrocephalus. Brainstem invasion often limits complete surgical excision. A whole-spine MRI scan is required to assess for drop metastasis.

Meningioma – a tumour that arises from arachnoid cap cells of the arachnoid villi in the meninges.

The WHO classification of meningiomas

Benign (Grade I) (90%)	Meningothelial, fibrous, transitional, psammomatous, angioblastic
Atypical (Grade II) (7%)	Choroid, clear cell, atypical
Anaplastic/malignant (Grade III) (2%)	Papillary, rhabdoid, anaplastic

Myoclonus – a brief, involuntary twitching of a muscle or a group of muscles.

Neuroenteric cyst – an intradural extramedullary cystic mass lined by gut endothelium.

Neurofibromatosis – an autosomal dominant disorder in which there is a risk of tumour formation in the brain. The disorder affects neural crest cells (e.g. Schwann cells, melanocytes and endoneurial fibroblasts). Cellular elements from these cell types proliferate throughout the body, forming tumours and disordered skin pigmentation.

Diagnostic criteria of neurofibromatosis type I

1. ≥6 café au lait macules >5 mm in greatest diameter in prepubertal individuals and >15 mm in greatest diameter in postpubertal individuals
2. ≥2 neurofibromas of any type or >1 plexiform neurofibroma
3. Freckling in the axillary or inguinal regions
4. Optic glioma
5. ≥2 Lisch nodules (iris hamartomas)
6. A distinctive osseous lesion, such as sphenoid dysplasia or thinning of the long bone cortex, with or without pseudoarthrosis
7. A first-degree relative (parent, sibling or offspring) with NF-1 according to the above criteria

Diagnostic criteria of neurofibromatosis type II

1. Bilateral vestibular schwannomas (VS) OR family history of NF-2 1 unilateral VS
   OR
   Any 2 of meningioma, glioma, neurofibroma, schwannoma, or posterior subcapsular lenticular opacities

Additional criteria

2. Unilateral VS plus any 2 of meningioma, glioma, neurofibroma, schwannoma, or posterior subcapsular opacities
   OR
3. Multiple meningioma (>2) plus unilateral VS OR any 2 of glioma, neurofibroma, schwannoma, or cataract

Normal pressure hydrocephalus – a condition characterized by a triad of cognitive impairment, gait disturbance and urinary incontinence. Intracranial pressure (ICP) measurements are not usually elevated.

Pain – a physiological response to noxious stimuli (e.g. thermal, mechanical, chemical and trauma) that are damaging to the underlying tissues.

Papilloedema – optic disc swelling that is caused by increased ICP. Fundoscopy may reveal venous engorgement, loss of venous pulsation, haemorrhages, blurring of optic margins or elevation of the optic disc. On visual field examination, there may be an enlarged blind spot. Visual acuity is normal until papilloedema has become advanced.

Parkinson's disease – a neurological syndrome characterized by tremor (resting, 4–7/seconds), cogwheel rigidity and bradykinesia. Other signs include postural instability, micrographia, mask-like facies or a festinating gait. It is a result of degeneration of pigmented dopaminergic neurons of the pars compacta of the substantia nigra, resulting in reduced levels of dopamine in the neostriatum (e.g. caudate nucleus, putamen, globus pallidus).

Rathke's cleft cyst – a benign, epithelium-lined intrasellar cyst found on the pituitary gland, which occurs when Rathke's pouch does not develop properly.

Modified Frisén scale for grading papilloedema

STAGE 0 – Normal optic disc or not a disc but no oedema/swelling

A. Prominence of the retinal nerve fiber layer at the nasal, superior and inferior poles in inverse proportion to disc diameter

B. Radial nerve fibre layer striations, without tortuosity

STAGE I – Minimal

A. C-shaped halo that is subtle and greyish with a temporal gap; obscures underlying retinal details

B. Disruption of normal radial NFL arrangement striations

C. Temporal disc margin normal

STAGE II – Low degree

A. Circumferential halo

B. Elevation – nasal border

C. No major vessel obscuration

STAGE III – Moderate

A. Obscuration of one or more segments of major blood vessels leaving disc

B. Circumferential halo

C. Elevation – all borders

D. Halo – irregular outer fringe with finger-like extensions

STAGE IV – Marked

A. Total obscuration on the disc of a segment of a major blood vessel on the disc

B. Elevation – whole nerve head, including the cup

C. Border obscuration – complete

D. Halo – complete

STAGE V – Severe

A. Partial obscuration of all vessels on disc and total obscuration of at least one vessel on disc

Scales and scoring systems

General

American Society of Anaesthesiologists' (ASA) classification.

Glasgow Coma Scale (GCS).

Glasgow Outcome Scale (GOS).

Evan's ratio for hydrocephalus.

Injury Severity Score (trauma).

Karnofsky Performance Status Scale.

Marshall's CT grading (trauma).

Modified Rankin scale.

Medical Research Council (MRC) grade for muscle power.

Functional

Ashworth scores for spasticity.

Engel's classification for epilepsy control following surgery.

Parkinson's Disability Score.

Oncology

Galassi classification for arachnoid cysts.

Glasscock–Jackson glomus tympanicum classification.

House–Brackmann grade of facial nerve function.

MacDonald criteria for determining tumour progression.

Simpson grades for extent of meningioma resection.

Spine

American Spinal Injury Association (ASIA) scores.

C1 fracture classification.

C1 fracture – Rule of Spence.

C2 hangman's fractures – modified Effendi system.

C2 odontoid fractures – Anderson and D'Alonzo classification.

Basilar Impression Measurements: McRae's line, Chamberlain's line, McGregor's line, Wackenheim's clivus-canal line,

Frankel grade.

Nurick's classification for cervical myelopathy.

Oswestry Disability Index.

Ranawat classification for neurological deficit.

Meyerding classification for spondylolisthesis.

Modic's classification for vertebral body marrow changes.

Patchell criteria for metastatic spinal cord compression.

Wiltse classification for spondylolisthesis.

Vascular

Barrow classification for congestive cardiac failure (CCF).

Burstein and Papile grading for neonatal intracranial haemorrhage.

Congard or Borden classification for dual arteriovenous fistula (DAVF).

Fisher grade for subarachnoid haemorrhage (SAH).

Hunt and Hess classification of SAH.

Modified Rankin Scale.

Pollock and Flickinger score for arteriovenous malformation (AVM) grading for radiosurgery.

Spetzler–Martin grade for AVMs.

World Federation of Neurosurgeons (WFNS) classification for SAH.

Peripheral nerves

Seddon's and Sunderland's classification of peripheral nerve injury.

Seizure – an abnormal paroxysmal cerebral neuronal discharge that results in alteration of sensation, motor function, behaviour or consciousness.

Syringomyelia – the development of a fluid-filled cavity or syrinx within the spinal cord. Several theories have been put forth to explain the pathogenesis of syringomyelia.

- **Gardner's hydrodynamic theory** – results from a 'water hammer'-like transmission of pulsatile CSF pressure via a communication between the fourth ventricle and the central canal of the spinal cord through the obex. There are craniospinal pressure differentials in the setting of fourth ventricular outlet obstruction; these differentials favour cerebrospinal fluid shifts from the fourth ventricle of the brain through the central canal of the spinal cord.

- **William's theory (craniospinal pressure dissociation)** – due to a differential between intracranial pressure and spinal pressure caused by a valve-like action at the foramen magnum by the tonsils. An increase in subarachnoid fluid pressure from increased venous pressure during coughing or a valsalva manoeuvre is localized to the intracranial compartment.

- **Oldfield's theory** – demonstrates that downward movement of the cerebellar tonsils during systole can be visualized with dynamic magnetic resonance imaging (MRI). This oscillation creates a piston effect in the spinal subarachnoid space that acts on the surface of the spinal cord and forces CSF through the perivascular and interstitial spaces into the syrinx, increasing intramedullary pressure. Signs and symptoms of neurological dysfunction that appear with distension of the syrinx are due to compression of long tracts, neurons and microcirculation. Symptoms referable to increased intramedullary pressure are potentially reversible by syrinx decompression.

	Resting tremor	Postural tremor	Action tremor
Description	Tremor when skeletal muscle is at rest.	Tremor when skeletal muscle holding in one position against gravity.	Tremor when in process of voluntary contraction of muscle.
Physical exam test	Observe at rest Observe while asking patient to do mental work (may increase).	Ask patient to extend arms and hold.	Finger to nose, rapid alternating movements or heel to shin.
Examples	Parkinson's disease, parkinsonian tremor (e.g. medications).	Essential tremor, increased physiologic tremor, Wilson's disease.	Cerebellar disease, multiple sclerosis, chronic alcohol abuse.

Tremor – an involuntary, rhythmical contraction of a muscle group, and can be classified into resting, postural or action tremor. There can be an overlap between the categories listed in the figure.

Trigeminal neuralgia – a condition characterized by unilateral sudden paroxysmal facial pain described as sharp, lancinating or shooting and lasting a few seconds, confined to the distribution of one or more branches of the trigeminal nerve (V2 and V3). Often the pain is triggered by sensory stimuli (e.g. brushing teeth or hair, talking and eating). The pathophysiology is related to the ephaptic transmission in the trigeminal nerve from large-diameter partially demyelinated A fibres to thinly myelinated A-delta and C (nociceptive) fibres. Differential diagnosis includes atypical facial pain, cluster headache, dental disease, orbital disease, sinusitis, giant cell arteritis, herpes zoster, temporomandibular joint (TMJ) dysfunction and intracranial tumour (e.g. posterior fossa).

Vascular malformation – a blood vessel abnormality. The vascular lesion can be classified as follows:

- AVM is a mesh of abnormal blood vessels characterized by the absence of normal interposing capillaries with no intervening brain parenchyma. As a result, oxygenated blood drains directly into the venous channel.

- Cavernous malformation – is an angiographically occult venous anomaly characterized by thin venous sinusoidal vessels with blood with no intervening brain matter. Its gross appearance resembles a mulberry.
- Capillary telangiectasia – is an angiographically occult vascular anomaly characterized by slightly enlarged capillaries with low flow with normal intervening brain parenchyma. They may be associated with Osler–Weber–Rendu syndrome (hereditary haemorrhagic telangiectasia).
- Venous angioma – is a tuft of abnormal medullary veins that converge into large central trunk and drain into either superficial or deep venous system. Intervening brain is present.

Vestibular schwannoma (acoustic schwannoma) – a benign intracranial extra-axial tumour that arises from the myelin-forming cells of the vestibulocochlear nerve.

Index